Other books in the Dx/Rx Oncology Series from Jones & Bartlett Learning

Dx/Rx:
Prostate Cancer

SECOND EDITION

Lewis J. Kampel, MD

Genitourinary Oncology Service
Department of Medicine
Sidney Kimmel Center for Prostate and Urologic Cancer
Memorial Sloan-Kettering Cancer Center and
   the Weill Cornell Medical College
New York, NY

Series Editor: Manish A. Shah, MD

Director of Gastrointestinal Oncology
Weill Cornell Medical College/New York–Presbyterian
   Hospital
New York, NY

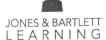

JONES & BARTLETT
L E A R N I N G

Jones & Bartlett Learning
5 Wall Street
Burlington, MA 01803
978-443-5000
info@jblearning.com
www.jblearning.com

Jones & Bartlett Learning books and products are available through most bookstores and onlir booksellers. To contact Jones & Bartlett Learning directly, call 800-832-0034, fax 978-443-800 or visit our website, www.jblearning.com.

Substantial discounts on bulk quantities of Jones & Bartlett Learning publications are available to corporations, professional associations, and other qualified organizations. For details and specific discount information, contact the special sales department at Jones & Bartlett Learning via the above contact information or send an email to specialsales@jblearning.com.

Dx/Rx: Prostate Cancer, Second Edition is an independent publication and has not been authorized, sponsored, or otherwise approved by the owners of the trademarks or service marks referenced in this product.

The authors, editor, and publisher have made every effort to provide accurate information. However, they are not responsible for errors, omissions, or for any outcomes related to the use of the contents of this book and take no responsibility for the use of the products and procedures described. Treatments and side effects described in this book may not be applicable to all people; likewise, some people may require a dose or experience a side effect that is not described herein. Drugs and medical devices are discussed that may have limited availability controlled by the Food and Drug Administration (FDA) for use only in a research study or clinical trial. Research, clinical practice, and government regulations often change the accepted standard in this field. When consideration is being given to use of any drug in the clinical setting, the health care provider or reader is responsible for determining FDA status of the drug, reading the package insert, and reviewing prescribing information for the most up-to-date recommendations on dose, precautions and contraindications, and determining the appropriate usage for the product. This is especially important in the case of drugs that are new or seldom used.

Production Credits

Executive Publisher: Christopher Davis
Associate Editor: Laura Burns
Production Assistant: Sarah Burke
Marketing Manager: Rebecca Rockel
Manufacturing and Inventory Control
    Supervisor: Amy Bacus

Composition: Jason Miranda, Spoke & Wheel
Cover Design: Kate Ternullo/Kristin Parker
Cover Image: © CLIPAREA | Custom media/ ShutterStock, Inc.
Printing and Binding: Malloy, Inc.
Cover Printing: Malloy, Inc.

Library of Congress Cataloging-in-Publication Data

Kampel, Lewis J.
  Dx/Rx. Prostate cancer / Lewis J. Kampel. — 2nd ed.
    p. ; cm.
  Prostate cancer
  Includes bibliographical references and index.
  ISBN-13: 978-0-7637-9453-8
  ISBN-10: 0-7637-9453-8
1. Prostate—Cancer—Handbooks, manuals, etc. I. Title. II. Title: Prostate cancer.
  [DNLM: 1. Prostatic Neoplasms—therapy—Handbooks. WJ 39]
  RC280.P7K36 2012
  616.99'463—dc23
                       2011028000
6048

Printed in the United States of America
16 15 14 13 12 10 9 8 7 6 5 4 3 2 1

#739835746

Dedication

This book is dedicated to the memory of my parents, Irving and Hannah Kampel.

Contents

Editor's Preface

Welcome to the Dx/Rx Oncology Series, a series of handbooks focusing on the practical management of common malignancies. *Dx/Rx: Prostate Cancer*, now in its second edition, provides a comprehensive overview of the diagnosis and management of prostate cancer. In recent years, the diagnosis and management of this disease have become considerably more complex, including a refinement of the Clinical States Model for disease management, the approval of several new drugs to treat advanced disease, and the emerging role of Robot Assisted Minimally Invasive Surgery. Prostate cancer is a diverse disease with variable natural history ranging from a prolonged, indolent disease course to an aggressive, shortened course associated with a high mortality rate. Treatment options for this disease are equally diverse and include surgery, brachytherapy, chemotherapy, and hormonal therapy. Fortunately, Dr. Kampel exceptionally integrates the nuances of the management of prostate cancer into this comprehensive and concise second edition of the *Dx/Rx: Prostate Cancer* handbook. The bulleted format, unique to this series, allows for quick access to vital and practical management issues for your patients' treatment. I know you will find this and several of the books in this series to be invaluable resources for your everyday use and patient care.

Manish A. Shah, MD

Preface to the First Edition

Adenocarcinoma of the prostate gland is the most commonly diagnosed nonskin cancer in men, and the second most common cause of cancer death in men. It is expected that in 2010, approximately 218,000 men will have been diagnosed with prostate cancer and approximately 32,000 men are expected to have died of this disease. Since 1992 and the advent of prostate-specific antigen (PSA) testing, approximately 86% of these cases are diagnosed with cancers limited to locoregional sites, allowing for high survival rates. Yet, many men go on to suffer morbidity and mortality as their prostate cancers recur.[1] Notably, although prostate cancer accounts to one third of all cancer diagnoses, it is responsible for only 10% of cancer deaths in men. The disparity is almost certainly a reflection of earlier diagnosis as a result of PSA testing (lead time bias) and the long natural history of this disease. However, the impact of treatment on the natural history of this cancer remains unclear.

The large volume of patients with prostate cancer who are expected to present themselves to urologists, radiation oncologists, medical oncologists, and primary care physicians creates a set of challenges as well as opportunities that are unique in cancer medicine. The challenges arise because we are asked to advise patients on a variety of treatment options without benefit of data that clearly distinguish among them in terms of superiority of outcome. Should I have a radical prostatectomy or radiotherapy? Open prostatectomy or laparoscopic? What about those seeds I read about in the paper? My PSA is going up; when should I start hormones? These are the questions all of us deal with every day in our clinical practices, but the answers are often unknown. The opportunity given to us by this huge cohort of patients is to learn from them, ideally by having them participate in clinical trials.

The purpose of this handbook is not to provide detailed arguments aimed at settling the large number of unanswered questions in this field. It is, instead, intended to be a practical guide to the current management of patients with prostate cancer. Because this is not a comprehensive textbook, it is impossible to include detailed analyses of, or even mention of, every last trial. Recommendations, when possible, are evidence based. On occasion, suggestions are made based on the clinical experience of the author or his colleagues. Every attempt possible is made to identify these as opinions. However, in this era of rapidly developing knowledge about prostate cancer and its management, it is incumbent upon the clinician to remain familiar with new literature that may impact his or her practice.

Lewis J. Kampel, MD

1. Jemal A, Siegel R, Xu J, Ward E. Cancer Statistics, 2010. CA Cancer J Clin. 2010;60:5 277–300.

Preface to the Second Edition

Even as the first edition of *Dx/Rx: Prostate Cancer* went to press, changes in the field of prostate oncology were already underway. In the 4 years since the original publication, advances have been made in many areas, both conceptual and practical. The concept of clinical states has been revised. More information has emerged about some of the genetic mechanisms that might lead to prostate cancer. New markers for diagnosis are under investigation. The role of adjunctive androgen-suppressive therapy for high-risk patients undergoing radiotherapy has been strengthened by a number of clinical trials. Randomized studies have shown that adjuvant radiotherapy offers a survival advantage for patients whose cancers are found to have extended beyond the prostate at time of prostatectomy. Several new agents (abiraterone acetate, MDV 3100) have shown promise for patients with advanced disease. And, a new drug (cabazitaxel) was found to improve survival in patients who have progressed through docetaxel.

At the same time, many of the questions raised in the first edition remain unanswered. Robotically Assisted Laparoscopic Prostatectomy (RALP) has become the most common type of prostatectomy, although there is no data demonstrating superiority over standard approaches. The battle over screening continues to rage, and the benefits of 5-alpha reductase inhibitors as preventative agents remain unclear despite 2 randomized studies.

The *Second Edition* describes and discusses these new developments and updates older ones. As always, the clinician must be aware that this is a rapidly changing field requiring close attention to the literature and clinical experience.

Lewis J. Kampel, MD

Acknowledgments

A number of people, over a lifetime, have contributed to the writing of this handbook, many in ways that they may never know. I would like to acknowledge my gratitude to Sidney Rosenfeld, a former teacher at Weequahic High School in Newark, NJ, for fostering my interest in biology and to the late Lester M. Goldman, MD, former director of laboratories at Newark Beth Israel Hospital, who gave me my first hospital job and stimulated my interest in hematology more than 45 years ago.

Special thanks to my family, Jan, Traci, and Jamie, for their support and encouragement and for putting up with me over the years during which this book was written and revised. And also, thanks to Claire for the calming effect that only felines can provide. I could not have accomplished this job without the support and advice of my colleagues at the Memorial Sloan Kettering Cancer Center, especially the members of the Genitourinary Oncology Service, the Department of Urology, and the Department of Radiation Oncology. Were it not for Dr. George Bosl, I would never have had the opportunity to write this book. I am grateful to Dr. Howard Scher for allowing me to develop an interest in prostate cancer, and for his work with Drs. Peter Scardino and James Eastham in creating a unique work environment that facilitates the interdisciplinary collaboration without which this book would not have been possible. Special thanks are in order to Drs. W. K. Kelly, Susan Slovin, Michael Morris, Dana Rathkopf, Daniel Danila, David Solit, David Shaffer, Farhang Rabbani, Fernando Bianco, Michael Zelefsky, Lanceford Chong, Marissa Kollmeier who contributed to the section on radiotherapy in Chapter 5, Victor Reuter, and Eugene Lind for providing material, reviewing the manuscript, and making helpful suggestions.

Finally, I would like to express my gratitude to all the patients with prostate cancer that I have had the privilege of treating. They have taught me far more than I could ever record in a book.

Lewis J. Kampel, MD

Notice

We have made every attempt to summarize accurately and concisely a multitude of references. However, the reader is reminded that times and medical knowledge change, transcription or understanding error is always possible, and crucial details can be omitted whenever such a comprehensive distillation as this is attempted in limited space. The primary purpose of this compilation is to cite literature on various sides of controversial issues; knowing where "truth" lies is usually difficult. We cannot, therefore, guarantee that every bit of information is absolutely accurate or complete. The reader should affirm that cited recommendations are reasonable still by reading the original articles and checking other sources, including local consultants as well as recent literature, before applying them.

Drugs and medical devices are discussed that may have limited availability controlled by the Food and Drug Administration (FDA) for use only in research study or clinical trial. The drug information presented has been derived from reference sources, recently published data, and pharmaceutical tests. Research, clinical practice, and government regulations often change the accepted standard in this field. When consideration is being given to use of any drug in the clinical setting, the clinician or reader is responsible for determining FDA status of the drug and reading the package insert and prescribing information for the most up-to-date recommendations on dose, precautions, and contraindications, and determining the appropriate usage for the product. This is especially important in the case of drugs that are new or seldom used.

Section I
Introduction

CHAPTER 1

Basic Principles

■ The Anatomy of the Prostate Gland[1]

The prostate is a small (20–25 g) exocrine gland located deep in the pelvis, interposed between the bladder and external urinary sphincter, surrounding the urethra. The bladder is located superiorally and anteriorally, and the rectum is located posteriorly. The cavernous nerves, critical for erection, run along its posterolateral surfaces on either side. **Figure 1-1** shows the prostate gland in relation to other pelvic structures. **Figure 1-2** details the surgical anatomy of the prostate gland, focusing on neurovascular structures.

The adult prostate gland is organized in a zonal fashion[2] (**Figure 1-3**).

- Transition zone
  - Surrounds urethra
  - Makes up 5% of glandular tissue of the prostate
  - Most common site for benign prostatic hypertrophy (BPH)
  - Only 15% of prostate cancers originate in the transition zone
- Central zone
  - Surrounds ejaculatory ducts
  - Makes up 20% of glandular tissue of the prostate
  - Prostate cancer rarely originates in the central zone
- Peripheral zone
  - Responsible for the bulk of prostate tissue
  - Makes up 70% of glandular tissue of the prostate
  - Most common site of origin of prostate cancer
  - Posterolateral location allows easy palpation by digital rectal exam

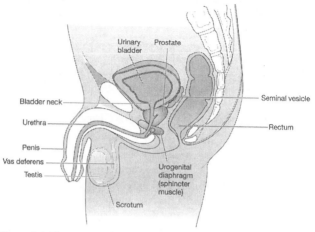

Figure 1-1 The prostate gland in relation to other pelvic structures. Adapted from image provided by James Eastham, MD, Medical Graphics.

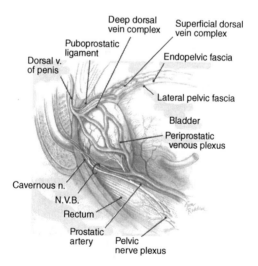

Figure 1-2 The surgical anatomy of the prostate gland. Reprinted from Ohori M and Scardino PT. Localized prostate cancer. *Curr Probl Surg.* 2002;39(9):833–957, with permission from Elsevier.

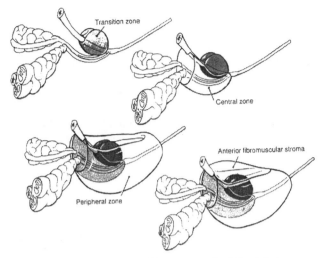

Figure 1-3 The zonal anatomy of the prostate gland. Reprinted with permission from McNeal JE, et al. Zonal Distribution of Prostatic Adenocarcinoma: Correlation with Histologic Pattern and Direction of Spread. *Am J Surg Pathol.* 1988;12(12):897–906.

- Anterior fibromuscular stroma
  - Nonglandular tissue
  - Forms what is commonly referred to as the capsule when the transition zone enlarges due to BPH

Function of the Prostate Gland

- Exact function of the prostate gland is not known
- Contributes seminal fluid to the ejaculate
- May promote sperm motility by secreting substances (prostate-specific antigen [PSA]) that liquefy the seminal coagulum

Incidence and Risk Factors

- Incidence
  - As discussed in the preface, prostate cancer is the most commonly diagnosed nonskin cancer in men, exceeding the frequency of cancers of the lung, breast, and colon. The expected death rate in men is second only to that of lung cancer[3] (**Table 1-1**).

- The incidence of prostate cancer increased dramatically between 1988 and 1992 as a result of the introduction of PSA testing. Between 1992 and 1995, the incidence rate dropped significantly as a result of the culling effect of PSA screening, before beginning to increase slowly and perhaps stabilizing in recent years.[3]

- Race
  - African American men continue to be at higher risk, both in terms of incidence and mortality (**Table 1-2**).
  - Black men from the Caribbean appear to have a risk of prostate cancer that is even higher than for African American men.[4]
  - Given these outcomes, it is not surprising that African American men present with higher PSA levels and higher Gleason scores. The extent to which this disparity is due to genetic versus social causes is not clear.[5]

Table 1-1 Estimated Incidence and Mortality Rates of Prostate Cancer Relative to Other Common Worldwide Malignancies

Cancer	Estimated New Cancer Cases in Men (2005)	Estimated Deaths in Men (2005)
Prostate	232,090	30,350
Lung	93,010	90,490
Colon	104,950	28,540

Table 1-2 Prostate Cancer Incidence and Mortality Rates by Race

Race	Incidence*	Death Rate*
All races	172.3	31.5
White	167.4	28.8
African American	271.3	70.4
Asian/Pacific Islander	100.7	13.0
American Indian/Alaskan Native	51.2	20.2
Hispanic/Latino	140.0	23.5

*Numbers are rates per 100,000 people.

- Age
  - Although prostate cancer remains a disease of the elderly, it does occur in men in their 40s.[6]
    - Incidence of prostate cancer in men between ages 40 and 59 years is 1 in 38.
    - Incidence of prostate cancer in men between ages 60 and 69 years is 1 in 14.
    - Incidence of prostate cancer in men over 70 is 1 in 7.
- Genetics
  - 85% sporadic
  - Familial prostate cancer: prostate cancer in one or more first-degree relatives
    - Lifetime risk of developing prostate cancer increases by:
      - A factor of 2 to 11, depending on the number of first-degree family members affected by the disease.[7]
      - Patients with a familial association of prostate cancer tend to develop the disease earlier in life.
      - Risk of prostate cancer increases if identical twin has disease but not if fraternal twin has disease.
  - Hereditary prostate cancer: prostate cancer inherited in a Mendelian fashion
    - Accounts for approximately 40% of all cases in men under the age of 55 years[8]
  - Gene changes associated with prostate cancer[8,9,10]
    - A number of genes have been associated with prostate cancer.
    - These genes tend to be involved in response to infection, inflammation or oxidative stress, or androgen receptor function.
    - Best known are:
      - RNASEL
      - MSR
      - SRD 5A2
    - Exact role and significance remain under investigation.
    - BRCA2[11]
      - Risk of prostate cancer three times normal among men who carry the BRCA2 mutation

- Men with BRCA2–associated prostate cancers are more likely to have higher grade disease, suffer recurrences, and die of prostate cancer than men with non-BRCA2 prostate cancer.
- Not associated with early-onset disease
- Several susceptibility loci under investigation on the first and the X chromosome
- Changes at 8q24 may be associated with the increased risk of prostate cancer seen in African American men[10]
- Single nucleotide polymorphisms (SNPs) at 8q24, 17q12, and 17q24.3 may increase overall risk by a factor of almost 10 depending on number of SNPs present[10]
- TMPRSS2-ERG
  - Fusion product of a PSA–regulated transmembrane serine protease gene and an erythroblastosis virus E26 sequence transcription factor
  - Present in 52% of prostate cancers[12]
  - Role in diagnosis and risk stratification under investigation
- A full discussion of the molecular and genetic changes linked to prostate cancer is beyond the scope of this handbook. The subject is well covered in several recent reviews.[8,10,12,13,14]
- Dietary factors[1,8]
  - The roles of several dietary factors remain under investigation as either promoting or inhibiting the development of prostate cancer.
  - Increased total fat, animal fat, and red meat intake have been associated with increased risk of prostate cancer.[15]
  - Vitamin D
    - Low levels associated with increased risk of prostate cancer
      - Known to induce differentiation in prostate cancer cells in vitro
      - May explain higher rates in northern latitudes
      - Studies attempting to correlate Vitamin D levels with the risk of developing prostate cancers have shown conflicting results. No prevention trials using Vitamin D have been published.[16]

- Plant estrogens
  - Plant estrogens such as genistein, found in soybeans, inhibit 5-alpha-reductase activity, in turn decreasing the levels of dihydroepitestosterone, the most potent ligand of the androgen receptor
- Antioxidants—potentially protective
  - Vitamin E
  - Selenium
    - Inverse relationship between selenium levels and risk of prostate cancer has been shown[17]
- Lycopenes
  - Potentially protective
- Factors not proven to be associated with increased risk of prostate cancer[1]
  - Cigarette smoking
  - Alcohol
  - Inflammation
  - Infection
  - Frequency of ejaculation
  - Vasectomy

■ Prevention of Prostate Cancer

The genetic, molecular, and epidemiologic factors alluded to earlier suggest opportunities for interventions aimed at lowering an individual's risk of developing prostate cancer. They can be divided into two categories: pharmacologic intervention and dietary/nutritional interventions.

- Pharmacologic intervention
  - Finasteride
    - In the Prostate Cancer Prevention Trial (PCPT), 18,882 men with no evidence of prostate cancer were randomly assigned to placebo or to finasteride, a potent 5-alpha-reductase inhibitor, for 7 years.[18]
    - Results
      - Prostate cancer was found in 18.4% of the finasteride group and in 24.4% of the control group ($p < .001$).
      - This amounts to a 24.8% reduction in prevalence over a 7-year period.
        - Reduction in risk limited to low grade (Gleason < 7) tumors

- Increased risk of higher grade tumors (Gleason 8–10)
  - RR 1.70 (95% CI 1.23–2.34)
- More sexual side effects but fewer urinary problems were seen in the finasteride group compared with the control group.
- Dutasteride
  - Reduction by Dutasteride of Prostate Cancer Events (REDUCE) Study[19]
    - 8231 men at high risk of prostate cancer randomized to dutasteride 5 mg per day versus placebo
      - Relative risk reduction is 22.8%
    - Biopsies done at 2 and 4 years
    - Statistically significant reduction in prostate cancer in dutasteride arm compared to placebo (19.9% vs 25.1%) p < 0.001
    - Reduction primarily in lower grade tumors
    - No reduction in risk of higher grade tumors (Gleason 7–10)
    - Increased risk of Gleason 8–10 cancers
      - RR 2.06 (95% CI 1.13–3.750)
    - Significant reduction in incidence of acute urinary retention in dutasteride arm (1.6% vs 6.7%) p = 0.01
    - Increased risk of heart failure in dutasteride arm (0.7% vs 0.4%) p = 0.03
    - Increased risk of loss of libido and erectile dysfunction on dutasteride arm
    - No difference in overall survival
    - No prostate cancer deaths
- *Comment:* The role of 5-alpha reductase inhibitors in the prevention of prostate cancer remains unclear. Concerns about increased risks of high-grade disease and lack of survival data hindered widespread acceptance of finasteride as a chemopreventive agent. The sexual side effects of these agents may make them less attractive to most men at low or average risk of prostate cancer. Further studies are needed to identify which patients are most likely to benefit from chemoprevention with either finasteride or dutasteride.

- Other agents under investigation:
  - Cyclooxygenase-2 (COX-2) inhibitors[20]
    - Anti-inflammatory agents may reduce oxidative stress leading to malignancy
  - Statins[21,22]
    - Preliminary evidence suggests that cholesterol-lowering drugs can reduce PSA, raising the possibility of employing them as prostate cancer preventive agents.
- Dietary and nutritional interventions
  - Vitamin E
    - The Alpha-Tocopherol, Beta-Carotene Cancer Prevention (ATBC) Trial[23]
    - This trial was designed to look for a reduction in lung cancer among smokers receiving alpha-tocopherol. A secondary analysis revealed a decrease in prostate cancer incidence and mortality in men receiving alpha-tocopherol.
    - A slight risk of hemorrhagic stroke was seen in the vitamin E arm among men with uncontrolled hypertension.
  - Selenium
    - In a randomized, double-blind trial, selenium 200 μg/day was shown to reduce the risk of prostate cancer by almost two thirds compared with control group values. These results were statistically significant (p = .002).[24]
    - A Southwest Oncology Group trial (SWOG 9917) looking at selenium as a preventive agent is currently underway.
  - The Selenium and Vitamin E Cancer Prevention Trial (SELECT)[25]
    - Randomized trial with almost 36,000 men to receive either selenium alone, vitamin E alone, a combination of selenium and vitamin E, or placebo. No significant difference in the rate of prostate cancer was found between any of the groups.
    - Nonsignificant increase in prostate cancer (p = 0.06) was seen in the vitamin E group.

* Tomato products and lycopenes
  * In vitro studies suggest that tomato powder, but not pure lycopene, reduced death from induced prostate cancer in rats.[26]

■ Prostate Cancer Screening

■ With the addition of PSA measurement to the digital rectal examination (see Chapter 2, pp. 23), the opportunity to diagnose prostate cancer in very early stages became realistic. Oncologic dogma suggests that finding cancer when the number of malignant cells is still small will result in a better chance of cure, because the likelihood of micrometastatic disease is diminished. In order for early detection to impact survival, the cancer must have lethal potential and be amenable to curative therapy.

■ Carcinoma of the prostate presents unique challenges in this regard. Although curative therapy (surgery and radiation) does exist, the lethality of prostate cancer varies and is difficult to predict in any given individual. Many men diagnosed with PSA–detected prostate cancer are not likely to die of the disease because of competing comorbidities, advanced age, or the indolent nature of their cancers. Further complicating the issue is the fact that potentially curative therapies for localized prostate cancer are also associated with a risk of permanent toxicities, such as incontinence or impotence.

■ In addition to tumor characteristics that may help distinguish potentially lethal prostate cancers from those that are not, patient factors have to be considered. For men of advanced age or with significant and fixed comorbidities, screening must be a carefully considered practice rather than a reflexive one, given the likelihood that some men will die of other diseases before their prostate cancer becomes an issue. On the other hand, some individuals are at higher risk for developing prostate cancer, and serious consideration must be given to screening for them.

- Perhaps a series of questions and answers will help clarify the issue.
  - Is prostate cancer a potentially lethal disease?
    - The answer is yes.
      - Albertsen et al. recently published an update with 20-year follow-up on 767 men with localized prostate cancer managed by observation alone or by hormone therapy.[27]
        - Although patients with low-grade prostate cancers (Gleason scores of 2–4) had a very low risk of dying of prostate cancer, the risk was higher among those with intermediate- and high-grade tumors (**Table 1-3**).
      - It is important to note that very few patients present with Gleason scores less than 6.
  - Are potentially curative therapies available?
    - The answer is yes (see Chapter 5, pp. 67).
  - Does screening detect prostate cancer in earlier stages?
    - The answer is yes.
      - Downward stage migration has been seen in the PSA era.
      - PSA-screened cancers are more likely to be organ-confined.[28]

Table 1-3 Risk of Death Stratified by Gleason Score

Gleason Score	Mortality Rate from Prostate Cancer*
2–4	6
5	12
6	30
7	65
8–10	121

*Per 1,000 person-years.

Data from Albertsen PC, Hanley JA, Fine J. 20-year outcomes following conservative management of clinically localized prostate cancer. *JAMA.* 2005;293:2095–2101.

- Is there an advantage to curative therapy?
    - The answer is yes.
        - The Scandinavian group updated the results of a randomized trial comparing radical prostatectomy with watchful waiting.[29]
            - This cohort of 695 patients had clinically localized well to moderately well differentiated disease, a reasonable life expectancy, and no serious comorbidity that would preclude radical prostatectomy.
            - At 10.8 years of follow-up there was improved overall prostate cancer-specific survival for patients undergoing prostatectomy:
                - At 12 years of follow-up, radical prostatectomy reduced the risk of death from prostate cancer by 35% (12.5% vs 17.9%, RR = 0.65, p = 0.03), but overall survival was not different, suggesting that beyond 10 years, competing comorbidities come into play.
                - It should be noted that many, if not all, of the patients entered on this trial had cancers that were not detected by PSA.
                - The risk of local progression and distant metastases was also significantly lower in the radical prostatectomy group.
    - Does prostate cancer screening save lives?
        - Two trials published in 2009 addressed but did not settle this issue.
            - The Prostate, Lung, Colorectal and Ovarian Cancer Screening Trial (PLCO)[30]
                - Randomly assigned 76,693 men to screening or "usual care" arms.
                - After 10 years of follow-up:
                    - Higher incidence in prostate cancer in screened arm (IRR 1.17, 95% C.I. 1.11–1.22)
                    - The death rate from prostate cancer was low (92 in screened arm vs. 82 in control arm)

- No difference observed between death rates from prostate cancer for screened versus not screened men RR 1.11 (95% CI 0.83–1.50)
- Problems included:
  - Short follow-up time
  - Many men (52%) in control arm had some screening.
- The European Randomized Study of Screening for Prostate Cancer (ERSPC)[31]
  - Randomized 182,160 European men aged 50–74 years
  - Subset core group of 162,387 men between the ages of 55–69
    - Screening versus no screening
    - Median follow-up of 9 years
    - No reduction in prostate cancer mortality for overall cohort
      - RR 0.85 (95% C.I. 0.73–1.00)
    - In the core group (ages 55–59) there was a 20% reduction in prostate cancer death in screened men (p = 0.04) RR 0.80 (95% C.I. 0.65–0.98)
      - When only those who actually underwent screening were evaluated, the reduction in prostate cancer death was even higher at 27%.
    - Positive effect of screening likely to increase with time

■ Conclusions

- The issue of screening for prostate cancer remains controversial, even as more and more sensitive techniques are being discovered to detect prostate cancer. Meanwhile there are still no good ways to distinguish tumors that need treatment from those likely to remain indolent.
- Guidelines from various organizations are rapidly changing and may differ in their recommendations.

- The following principles would seem reasonable at the time of this edition:
  - For men with advanced age or life-limiting comorbidities, screening for prostate cancer will probably not be beneficial. Yet, the current medicolegal climate makes it advisable to discuss screening with those patients and to document that discussion.
  - For younger and healthier men, the pros and cons of screening should be discussed and documented.
  - Men who are at higher risk by virtue of family history, known genetic predisposition, or African American/Caribbean ancestry should be offered screening at younger ages, perhaps beginning at age 40 years.

■ Prostate Cancer Clinical States and Transitions

- The universe of prostate cancer encompasses a large cohort of men with different issues that present themselves at different times in the course of the disease.
  - For men who are at risk (any man over the age of 40 years), the major issues may be prevention, screening, and early diagnosis.
  - The choice of treatment and the quality of life problems that result are the concerns of newly diagnosed men.
  - For men with recurrent disease, prolongation of life and palliation become paramount.
- The concept of prostate cancer clinical states and transitions allows clinicians to better visualize the changing prognosis, goals, and therapeutic objectives at different time points in their patients' disease.[32]
  - **Figure 1-4** graphically displays this concept. Patients remain in one clinical state until they move on (or progress) to the next one.
    - The clinical states are generally self-explanatory.
      - Men in the no cancer diagnosis, localized disease, or rising PSA state can either die of nonprostate cancer causes or move on to the next state.
        - Death from prostate cancer does not occur while patients are in these states.

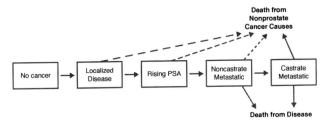

- -▶ Pathways from a clinical state to a non-prostate cancer related mortality
—▶ Pathways from a clinical state to a prostate cancer related mortality

Figure 1-4 Prostate clinical states. Adapted from Scher HI, et al. *Urology.* 2000;55(3):323–327, with permission from Elsevier.

- Men in the noncastrate-resistant or castrate-resistant (hormone refractory) state will go on to die of their prostate cancer unless they die of another illness.
- It is important to remember that the patient stays in one clinical state until he progresses to the next. Thus, the patient with overt metastatic disease who has never been treated for advanced disease with androgen deprivation therapy is considered to be in the noncastrate-resistant state. He remains in that state from the time that androgen deprivation therapy is started until his disease becomes hormone refractory. At that point he enters the castrate-resistant state.

■ References

1. Scher HI, Leibel SA, Fuks Z, Cordon-Cardo C, Scardino PT, et al. Prostate cancer. In: DeVita VT, Hellman S, Rosenberg SA, eds. *Cancer: Principles and Practice of Oncology,* 7th ed. Philadelphia: Lippincott, Williams and Wilkins; 2005:1192–1259.
2. Wheeler TM. Anatomy and pathology of prostate cancer. In: Vogelzang NJ, ed. *Comprehensive Textbook of Genitourinary Oncology.* Baltimore: Williams and Wilkins; 1996:621–639.
3. Jemal A, Siegel R, Ward E, et al. Cancer statistics, 2009. *Cancer J Clin.* 2009;59:225–249.
4. Glover FE Jr, Coffey DS, Douglas LL, Cadogan M, Russell H, Tulloch T, et al. The epidemiology of prostate cancer in Jamaica. *J Urol.* 1998; 159: 1984–1987.

5. Cooperberg MR, Park S, Carroll PR. Prostate cancer 2004: insights from national disease registries. *Oncology.* 2004;18:1239–1247.

6. American Cancer Society. Cancer Facts and Figures 2006. American Cancer Society; 2006. www.cancer.org/downloads/STT/CAFF2006 PW secured.pdf.

7. Steinberg GD, Carter BS, Beaty TH, et al. Family history and the risk of prostate cancer. *Prostate.* 1990;17:337–347.

8. Deutsch E, Maggiorella L, Eschwege P, et al. Environmental, genetic, and molecular features of prostate cancer. *Lancet Oncol.* 2004;5:303–313.

9. Garber JE, Offit K. Heriditary cancer predisposition syndromes. *J Clin Oncol.* 2005;23:276–292.

10. Patel AR, Klein EA. Risk factors for prostate cancer. *Nat Clin Pract Urol.* 2009; 6:2, 87–95.

11. Gallagher DJ, Gaudet MM, Pal P, et al. Germline BRCA Mutations denote a clinicopathological subset of prostate cancer. *Clin Cancer Res.* 2010;16(7):2115–2121.

12. Kumar-Sinha C, Tomlins SA, Chinnaiyan AM. Recurrent gene fusions in prostate cancer. *Nat Rev Cancer.* 2008; 8(7): 497–511.

13. Nelson WG, De Marzo AM, Isaacs WB. Prostate cancer. *N Engl J Med.* 2003;349:366–381.

14. Shaffer DR, Scher HI. Prostate cancer: a dynamic illness with shifting targets. *Lancet Oncol.* 2003;4:407–414.

15. Giovannucci E, Rimm EB, Colditz GA, et al. A prospective study of dietary fat and risk of prostate cancer. *J Natl Cancer Inst.* 1993;85:1571–1579.

16. Trottier G, Bostrom PJ, Lawrentschuk N, Fleshner NE. Nutraceuticals and prostate cancer prevention: a current review. *Nat Rev Urol.* 2010;7:21–30.

17. Li H, Stampfer MJ, Giovannucci EL, et al. A prospective study of plasma selenium levels and prostate cancer risk. *J Natl Cancer Inst.* 2004;96:696–703.

18. Thompson IM, Goodman PJ, Tangen CM, et al. The influence of finasteride on the development of prostate cancer. *N Engl J Med.* 2003;349:215–224.

19. Andriole GL, Bostwick DG, Brawley OW, et al. Effect of dutasteride on the risk of prostate cancer. *N Engl J Med.* 2010;362:1192–1202.

20. Canby-Hagino ED, Thompson IM. Mechanisms of disease: prostate cancer—a model for cancer chemoprevention in clinical practice. *Nat Clin Pract Oncol.* 2005;2:255–261.

21. Moyad MA. Why a statin and/or another proven heart healthy agent should be utilized in the next major cancer chemoprevention trial: part II. *Urol Oncol.* 2004;22:472–477.

22. Moyad MA. Why a statin and/or another proven heart healthy agent should be utilized in the next major cancer chemoprevention trial: part I. *Urol Oncol.* 2004;22:466–471.

23. The Alpha-Tocopherol, Beta Carotene Cancer Prevention Study Group. The effect of vitamin E and beta carotene on the incidence of lung cancer and other cancers in male smokers. *N Engl J Med.* 1994;330:1029–1035.

24. Clark LC, Dalkin B, Krongrad A, et al. Decreased incidence of prostate cancer with selenium supplementation: results of a double-blind cancer prevention trial. *Br J Urol.* 1998; 81:730–734.

25. Lippman SM, Klein EA, Goodman PJ. Effect of selenium and vitamin E on risk of prostate cancer and other cancers. The Selenium and Vitamin E Cancer Prevention Trial (SELECT). *JAMA.* 2009; 301(1); 39–51.

26. Boileau TW, Liao Z, Kim S, et al. Prostate carcinogenesis in N-methyl-N-nitrosourea (NMU)-testosterone-treated rats fed tomato powder, lycopene, or energy-restricted diets. *J Natl Cancer Inst.* 2003;95:1578–1586.

27. Albertsen PC, Hanley JA, Fine J. 20-year outcomes following conservative management of clinically localized prostate cancer. *JAMA.* 2005;293:2095–2101.

28. National Comprehensive Cancer Network. Prostate cancer early detection clinical practice guidelines in oncology. *JNCCN.* 2004;2:190–207.

29. Bill-Axelson A, Holmberg L, Filen L, et al. Radical prostatectomy versus watchful waiting in localized prostate cancer: The Scandinavian Prostate Cancer Group 4 Randomized Trial. *JNCI.* 2008;100(16):1144–1154.

30. Andriole GL, Reding D, Grubb RL, et al. Mortality results from a randomized prostate-cancer screening trial. *NEJM.* 2009;360:1310–1319.

31. Schroder FH, Hugosson J, Roobol MJ, et al. Screening and prostate-cancer mortality in a randomized European study. *NEJM* 2009;360:1320–1328.

32. Scher HI, Heller G. Clinical states in prostate cancer: toward a dynamic model of disease progression. *Urology.* 2000;55:323–327.

Section II
Clinical State: No Cancer Diagnosis

CHAPTER 2

The Diagnosis of Prostate Cancer

■ Introduction

- The sine qua non of any cancer diagnosis is still based on the careful evaluation of an adequate biopsy specimen by an experienced pathologist.

- In the case of prostate cancer, the decision to perform a biopsy is usually based on digital rectal examination of the prostate and/or the level of prostatic-specific antigen in the blood.

- This chapter discusses the diagnosis of prostate cancer from the classical point of view: symptoms (history), physical examination, laboratory data, imaging, and biopsy.

■ History

- Since the widespread implementation of prostate-specific antigen (PSA) screening as a means of detecting early prostate cancer, most men diagnosed with prostate cancer are asymptomatic.

- Although many who are ultimately diagnosed with prostate cancer initially seek urologic evaluation for a variety of complaints, their symptoms are generally coincidental to the cancer diagnosed after an elevated PSA level is found.

- Symptoms that may or may not be related to early prostate cancer
  - Erectile dysfunction or loss of libido
  - Nocturia, frequency, hesitancy, or urgency
  - Dysuria or urinary tract infection
  - Hematospermia
  - Perineal or scrotal discomfort

- Although any of those symptoms can be associated with more advanced locoregional disease, they are more often caused by unrelated processes such as benign prostatic hypertrophy (BPH), urinary tract infection, and prostatitis, or by a variety of other benign conditions.
- Despite the widespread use of the PSA determination, some men still present with more advanced locoregional disease or even widespread metastatic disease. Many of them are also asymptomatic, but certain symptoms are more worrisome.
  - Symptoms of advanced locoregional prostate cancer
    - Bulky prostate tumors can cause any of the symptoms described for early prostate cancers.
    - Invasion of the neurovascular bundle can cause erectile dysfunction.
    - Involvement of pelvic nerve roots can cause severe pain in the perineum or gluteal area.
    - Bladder invasion can result in hematuria or renal failure due to ureteral obstruction.
      - Locally advanced prostate cancers may cause outflow obstruction and urinary retention.
      - Posterior growth of the tumor into the rectal lumen can cause constipation, tenesmus, or even frank rectal obstruction.
- Surprisingly, many patients with prostate cancer still present with disseminated disease. Their symptoms may be of a general nature (anorexia, weight loss, fatigue), or they may suggest specific metastatic sites.
  - Symptoms of metastatic prostate cancer
    - Bone pain due to skeletal metastases is the most common symptom of metastatic prostate cancer.
    - Massive involvement of para-aortic or retroperitoneal lymph nodes may cause back pain, ureteral obstruction, or lymphedema of the lower extremities and genitals.
    - Bone marrow replacement can cause fatigue or dyspnea due to anemia, or bleeding due to thrombocytopenia. Significant neutropenia in the un-treated patient is rare.

- Inappropriate activation of the blood coagulation system can manifest itself as either generalized bleeding due to disseminated intravascular coagulation (DIC) or thromboembolic phenomena due to a hypercoagulable state. (*Note*: DIC is occasionally seen after biopsy of the prostate or of a metastatic site.)
- Neurologic symptoms can include lower extremity weakness due to spinal cord compression, cranial nerve palsies due to base of skull involvement, and facial numbness due to involvement of cranial nerve foramina.

■ General Physical Examination

- The general physical examination is an important part of the overall assessment of the patient with suspected prostate cancer. Findings concerning the overall health status of the patient and significant comorbidities are important in planning treatment after the diagnosis is made and may affect the decision whether or not to pursue the diagnosis at all. The general physical examination may also yield signs that suggest advanced or disseminated disease. Specific attention should be paid to lymph node bearing areas, particularly in the supraclavicular region. The documentation of a baseline neurologic exam will be appreciated later in the course of the disease, when subtle neurologic changes may be otherwise difficult to interpret.

■ Digital Rectal Examination (DRE)

- Because the prostate is located low in the pelvis and immediately anterior to the thin-walled rectum, the DRE has the potential to be a safe and inexpensive way of diagnosing prostate cancer. Several factors limit its usefulness:
  - Subjectivity of the examination, operator dependence, limited patient tolerance, and inability to detect microscopic disease result in low sensitivity and specificity.

- Even though most prostate cancers develop in the peripheral zone, and thus should be easily appreciated by DRE, some occur in the transitional zone, which is more difficult to palpate. Yet, in combination with the PSA, this exam remains an integral part of the evaluation of a patient with suspected or proven prostate cancer.
- In order to obtain the most information from this examination, patient cooperation and comfort are mandatory.
  - Technique of DRE
    - The DRE should be performed in a location where the patient's privacy is assured. Family members and other visitors should be asked to leave the room unless otherwise requested by the patient.
    - The patient should be allowed to visit the bathroom before the examination.
    - The patient should be properly positioned, either
      - standing on the floor with elbows on the table and feet brought close to the table edge, or
      - in the left lateral decubitus position (if the examiner is right-handed) or on his right side if the examiner is left-handed.
    - The examiner should glove both hands (trust me on this one).
    - Adequate lubricant should be applied to the examining glove.
    - Gentle pressure should be applied to the anal opening before insertion of finger ("always knock before entering").
    - Radial traction on the anal ring should be avoided.
    - The prostate should be carefully palpated for nodules, consistency, and size.
    - The examiner's finger should sweep from side to side in order to appreciate the lateral sulci and any obvious extension of the tumor beyond the prostate itself.
    - Asking the patient to perform a Valsalva maneuver may allow more thorough examination of the prostate base.

- ▪ The entire circumference of the rectum should be examined to rule out other pathology.
- ▪ Materials needed to allow the patient to clean up after the examination should be available.
- The normal prostate should be smooth, regular, and without nodularity. DRE findings that suggest malignancy include:
  - ▪ A discrete hard nodule
  - ▪ A less discrete area of induration
  - ▪ Diffuse induration of the prostate often with a "pebbly" consistency
  - ▪ A massively enlarged, "rock-hard" prostate protruding into the rectal lumen
- However, in the PSA era, most patients have a normal DRE or findings consistent with BPH.
- ▪ The decision to biopsy
  - Any suspicious DRE finding should trigger consideration of a prostate biopsy, notwithstanding the PSA value.
  - At the time of DRE, it should be remembered that very high grade, poorly differentiated prostate cancers may not express PSA, and thus the serum PSA level may be misleadingly low.
  - For patients of very advanced age and for those with serious comorbidities, the decision to perform a biopsy of the prostate becomes more complex.
  - If the patient is not a candidate for definitive or even palliative therapy, the value of performing a biopsy is questionable.
  - On the other hand, assuming there are no contraindications to biopsy such as anticoagulation or a bleeding disorder, transrectal biopsy is a relatively simple outpatient procedure. The information obtained may be worthwhile in making overall management decisions, even if no specific cancer treatment will be offered.

■ PSA

■ PSA is a serine protease member of the human tissue kallikrein family that is useful in the initial diagnosis of prostate cancer and for following response to therapy. Its function is to liquefy the ejaculate in order to increase sperm motility and facilitate conception.

■ Synthesis of PSA[1]

* PSA is produced primarily by ductal and acinar epithelial cells of the prostate gland. Small amounts of PSA from perianal and periurethral glands, the breasts, the thyroid, and the placenta do not contribute to measurable PSA in the blood.

* Transcription of the PSA gene is regulated by the androgen receptor (AR). When AR function is suppressed, as in androgen-suppressive therapy, PSA decrease may be due to decreased AR stimulation rather than, or in addition to, reduction in tumor volume.

* Consequently, reduction in PSA values may not accurately correlate with antitumor response, particularly in the androgen-independent state.

* The initial protein, preproPSA, contains a 17-amino acid leader sequence. ProPSA (inactive) is formed when the leader sequence is cleaved off. Active PSA is formed when a 7-amino acid sequence is cleaved from the N-terminal end of proPSA.

* Normally, a small amount of active PSA gains access to the circulation, where it is bound and inactivated by alpha-antichymotrypsin (ACT). This is measured as bound PSA.

* In the lumen, active PSA is inactivated by proteolysis.

* The inactive product, PSA, gains access to the bloodstream, where it circulates as free PSA.

* In prostate cancer, disruption of the basement membrane results in leakage of proPSA into the bloodstream (measured as bound PSA), leaving less proPSA to be converted to active PSA in the lumen and, consequently, less active PSA to be inactivated and circulate as free PSA.

- The net result is an increase in total PSA levels and a decrease in free PSA levels compared with normal, a fact that can be exploited for diagnostic purposes (**Figure 2-1**).
- Various PSA and proPSA isoforms, including complexed PSA and so-called benign or transitional zone PSA, are currently under investigation to determine their value in discriminating between prostate cancer and BPH.

■ Normal PSA values
- Choosing a normal value for PSA, above which biopsy should be performed, has important ramifications.
  - ■ Too high a value results in significant cancers being missed.
  - ■ On the other hand, a value set too low increases the number of unnecessary biopsies and leads to the detection of cancers with unknown biologic significance.
  - ■ Until recently, the generally accepted upper limit for normal levels was 4 ng/ml. Above this level, the likelihood of having a positive biopsy is 30–35%.[2] When the PSA level is ≥ 10 ng/ml, the risk of finding prostate cancer is as high as 60%.

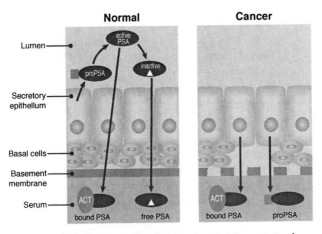

Figure 2-1 PSA synthesis and binding. Reprinted with permission from the American Society of Clinical Oncology. Balk SP, et al. *J. Clin Oncol.* 2003;21:383–391.

- Significant prostate cancer can be found at lower PSA levels. Among men with PSA values less than 4.0 ng/ml enrolled in the Prostate Cancer Prevention Trial (PCPT), 15% were found to have prostate cancer, of which 15% were high grade.[3]
  - **Table 2-1** summarizes the findings for patients with PSA values from less than 0.5 to 4.0 ng/ml. Although this study does not address the benefit of early diagnosis of cancers found at this PSA level, between 10% and 25% of cancers found were high grade.
  - Based on this report, many clinicians now use a PSA level of 2.5 ng/ml as the lower limit of normal.
- Other authors have suggested age-specific PSA normals:[4]

Age	PSA (ng/ml)
40–49	< 2.5
50–59	< 3.5
60–69	< 4.5
70–79	< 6.5

- Confounding factors
  - Factors that increase PSA
    - BPH
      - 20% of patients with BPH have PSA levels between 4 and 10 ng/ml.
      - 3% have PSA levels greater than 10 ng/ml.
    - Prostate biopsy and TURP can increase PSA levels for 6 weeks.
    - Prostatic massage and ejaculation can increase PSA levels for 2–3 days.
    - Prostatitis
      - PSA should be repeated after a full course of antibiotic therapy.
  - Factors that decrease PSA
    - Finasteride and other 5-alpha reductase inhibitors
      - Finasteride is a 5-alpha-reductase inhibitor commonly used in the treatment of obstructive symptoms due to BPH and male pattern baldness.

Table 2-1 Relationship of the Prostate-Specific Antigen (PSA) Level to the Prevalence of Prostate Cancer and High-Grade Disease*

PSA Level	No. of Men (N = 2950)	Men with Prostate Cancer (N = 449)	Men with High-Grade Prostate Cancer (N = 67)	Sensitivity	Specificity
		No. of Men (%)	No./Total No. (%)		
≤ 0.5 ng/ml	486	32 (6.6)	4/32 (12.5)	1.0	0.0
0.6–1.0 ng/ml	791	80 (10.1)	8/80 (10.0)	0.93	0.18
1.1–2.0 ng/ml	998	170 (17.0)	20/170 (11.8)	0.75	0.47
2.1–3.0 ng/ml	482	115 (23.9)	22/115 (19.1)	0.37	0.80
3.1–4.0 ng/ml	193	52 (26.9)	13/52 (25.0)	0.12	0.94

*High-grade disease was defined by a Gleason score of 7 or greater. The population was restricted to men with a PSA level of 4.0 ng per milliliter or less throughout the study. Therefore, the definitions of sensitivity and specificity are restricted to cutoff values of less than 4.0 ng per milliliter (the cutoff values are equal to the lower value of the ranges in the PSA column [0.0, 0.6, 1.1, 2.1, and 3.1 ng/ml]). Sensitivity was defined as the proportion of men with cancer who had a PSA value about the cutoff among all men with cancer who had a PSA value of 4.0 ng per milliliter or less. Specificity was defined in a like manner.

Reprinted with permission from Thompson IM, et al. Prevalence of prostate cancer among men with a prostate-specific antigen level. *N Engl J Med* 2004;350:2239–46.

- After 6 months of therapy, PSA values may be reduced 35% to more than 60%.[2] However, it should be emphasized that the effect of finasteride on serum PSA levels is highly variable.
  - Supplements
    - Over-the-counter herbal supplements used for urinary symptoms may contain plant alkaloids with estrogenic activity that suppresses PSA levels.
- High-grade or neuroendocrine cancers may not express PSA.
- There is no evidence that DRE significantly increases PSA.
- Improving the sensitivity/specificity of PSA levels
  - Percent free PSA (see synthesis of PSA on page 28)
    - The fraction of free or unbound PSA in the blood is decreased in prostate cancer.
    - Value useful primarily in patients with negative DRE and PSA less than 10 ng/ml
      - If a free PSA level of less than 25% were used to trigger biopsy consideration, 90% of cancers would be detected, and unnecessary biopsies would be reduced by 20%.[5]
  - Complexed PSA (cPSA)
    - cPSA assays primarily measure PSA-ACT complexes.[6]
      - For patients with total PSA values between 2.5 and 4.0 ng/ml, a cPSA level of greater than 2.2 ng/ml enhances prostate cancer detection compared with the use of percent free PSA. Measuring cPSA density, and more specifically cPSA density in the transitional zone, may be even better with the caveats mentioned in the following section.
  - PSA density
    - This value is calculated by dividing the serum PSA level by the prostate volume as determined by ultrasound.
    - Levels greater than or equal to 0.15 mg/ml/cc are considered abnormal. Because the measurement of prostate volume by ultrasound is not highly reproducible, PSA density is not commonly used.

- PSA velocity
  - This is the rate at which the PSA level increases with time.
  - Using a cutoff of 0.75 ng/ml/year increased sensitivity for patients whose PSA levels were less than 4.0 ng/ml.
- PCA3[7]
  - A highly overexpressed gene in prostate cancer cells compared to normal cells
    - Located at 9 q21–22
    - Found in 95% of primary prostate cancers
    - Initially named differential display clone 3
  - Current techniques use transcription-mediated amplification to measure PCA3 mRNA in urine and compare it with PSA mRNA, creating a PCA3 score (ratio of PCA3 mRNA to PSA mRNA)
  - Appears to be more sensitive and more specific than serum PSA in predicting a positive biopsy when PCA score is > 35
  - May be useful in
    - Initial diagnosis
    - Predicting outcomes of repeat biopsy in patients with high risk but initial negative biopsy
    - Distinguishing high-risk from low-risk cancers and thus allowing watchful waiting with more comfort
  - Combining PCA3 score with other markers such as TMPRSS2–ERG fusion may enhance sensitivity and specificity
  - Exact role of this test remains unclear at the time of this edition
- Other biomarkers
  - Various biomarkers and combination of biomarkers are currently under investigation including multiple isoforms of PSA and other kallikreins including free, complexed, and intact PSA as well as human kallikrein 2.[8]

■ Transrectal Ultrasonography (TRUS)

■ Insufficient sensitivity and specificity when used alone

■ Detection of smaller, nonpalpable lesions by PSA level limits usefulness of TRUS in diagnosing cancer

■ May be useful in estimating prostate gland volume in order to plan radiotherapy

■ Diagnostic value when used to calculate PSA density is questionable

■ Major use is in guiding prostate biopsy

■ Indications for TRUS–Guided Biopsy

■ Even in younger, healthier men, the decision should not be a reflexive one. Many of the cancers found may not be significant, but anxiety over unpredictable outcomes often leads to intervention that can be dangerous or result in a negative effect on quality of life.

■ On the other hand, prostate biopsy is relatively safe, and even the very elderly might benefit from palliative androgen-suppressive therapy.

■ Finally, there is something to be said for knowing the diagnosis, should the cancer spread and become symptomatic in the future. Before a PSA level is obtained and again before a biopsy is performed, the advantages and disadvantages should be discussed in detail with the patient.

■ Prostate biopsy should be *considered* in the following circumstances, assuming there are no contraindications and the patient is likely to benefit from either palliative or potentially curative therapy.

  * Positive DRE regardless of PSA level
    ■ Distinct nodule
    ■ Large, rock-hard, irregular prostate
    ■ Suspicious induration
    ■ Abnormal (high) age specific PSA (see page 30)
  * Percent free PSA level of less than 25%
  * Complexed PSA level of greater than 2.2 ng/ml
  * PSA velocity of greater than 0.75 ng/ml/year
  * The threshold for biopsy should be lower for African American and Caribbean men and for men with a strong family history of prostate cancer.

■ TRUS–Guided Biopsy

- The decision to perform a biopsy of the prostate gland is a complex one that should take into consideration a number of factors beyond the patient's PSA level and DRE findings. The axiom that no test should be performed unless the results will change management is as important in this setting as it is anywhere in medicine.

- For men with very advanced age or a serious comorbidity for whom life expectancy is short, making a diagnosis of early prostate cancer is unlikely to change either quality of life or survival.

- Biopsy performed with a spring-loaded gun, using transrectal ultrasonography to guide path

- Patients should be off antiplatelet agents, aspirin, and nonsteroidal anti-inflammatory agents for 1–2 weeks prior to the procedure.

- Patients on warfarin should stop that agent well enough in advance to allow the international normalized ratio (INR) to drop to safe levels before the biopsy is performed.

- Patients who cannot tolerate more than transient cessation of anticoagulation can be "bridged" with the use of either unfractionated or low-molecular-weight heparin before and after the procedure.

- Prophylactic antibiotics are generally ordered prior to the procedure.
  - Endocarditis prophylaxis should be considered for high-risk patients, such as those with valvular heart disease or artificial valves.

- Complications[4,9]
  - Pain, which may be averted with local anesthesia
  - Sepsis
  - Urinary retention
    - More likely with large biopsy numbers (> 13 cores)
    - Increased risk if urethra is violated
  - Bleeding–usually mild and self-limiting
    - Hematuria (13–80%)
    - Hematospermia (5–89%)
    - Hematochezia (2.4–37%)

- Disseminated intravascular coagulation[10] can be triggered by biopsy of the prostate, but this complication is rare.

■ TRUS Biopsy—Sampling[11]

- Prostate biopsy techniques have evolved with the development of spring-loaded biopsy needles. The goal is to develop techniques that increase the sensitivity of the test without increasing the complication rate.
- Initial techniques involved performing a biopsy of palpable or sonographically suspicious abnormalities.
- Since the advent of PSA detection, most cancers are not palpable and are not sonographically detectable.
  - Sextant biopsy
    - Tissue samples from the base, apex, and mid-zone of each side of the prostate
    - Higher yield than biopsy of sonographically detected lesions alone
    - Transitional zone not sampled
    - 20–40% false-negative rate
  - Extended biopsy
    - Sampling of increased numbers of cores improves cancer detection rates.
    - Although the optimal number of biopsy cores is not known, current National Comprehensive Cancer Network (NCCN) guidelines recommend a biopsy scheme that obtains 10–12 samples from the peripheral zone, including the lateral horns.
  - Transitional zone (TZ) biopsy
    - The yield from TZ biopsy among men with negative sextant biopsy results is only 9–15%.[12]
    - Thus, TZ biopsy is not generally included in the initial biopsy scheme.
- The pathology of prostate cancer when the histologic diagnosis is unequivocal is discussed in the next chapter.

- The prostate biopsy results may occasionally be nondiagnostic—suspicious but inconclusive for cancer.
  - These biopsy specimens may contain an insufficient number of suspicious glands for diagnosis, or they may reveal atypical small acinar proliferation (ASAP) or high-grade prostatic intraepithelial neoplasia (PIN).
  - In some cases, the clinical suspicion of cancer based on either the PSA level or the DRE results is sufficiently high that a negative initial biopsy result does not allay those fears.
  - Any of these circumstances might trigger a repeat biopsy.

■ Repeat Prostate Biopsy

- Although current biopsy techniques have improved, false-negatives still occur.
- Repeat biopsies are indicated in men with negative initial biopsy results and increasing PSA levels or PSA levels that are higher than expected for the patient's age and prostate size.
- Positive results of second biopsies are more common after negative sextant biopsy results (29–36%) than after negative extended scope biopsy results (9–10%).
- Repeat biopsies may also be indicated when the biopsy is inconclusive or when ASAP is found.
- Some clinicians recommend repeat biopsy within a year for patients with high-grade PIN, particularly if it is seen in three or more cores.
- The optimal timing of repeat prostate biopsy remains unclear.
  - Repeat biopsies should be done with the extended scope technique and should include at least one transitional zone sample.

■ ASAP[11]

- Presence of atypical glands lacking definitive features of malignancy
- High-molecular-weight cytokeratin (34βE12) (HMWCK) staining needed for diagnosis
  - Positive staining indicates intact basal membrane consistent with ASAP.

- Negative stain indicates disruption of basal membrane and is diagnostic of cancer
  - P63 is a nuclear protein that may be a better marker for prostatic basal cells then HMWCK.[13]
  - Alpha-methylacyl-CoA racemase (P504S)(AMACR) is a useful histochemical marker for prostate cancer.[14]
    - 80–100% of prostate cancers stain positive for AMACR.[13]
    - PIN may also stain positive for AMACR.
- Combination of negative staining for HMWCK and P63 associated with positive staining for AMACR in otherwise equivocal situations strongly supports diagnosis of cancer.
- Positive staining for HMWCK or P63 and negative staining for AMACR supports diagnosis of ASAP.
  - The finding of ASAP in initial biopsy result is associated with a higher risk (30–60%) of finding cancer on subsequent biopsy result after both initial sextant and extended scope biopsies.
  - Thus, the finding of ASAP should be followed by repeat biopsy.

■ High-Grade PIN (HGPIN)[11]

- HGPIN refers to groups of atypical cells lining normal prostatic acini.
  - Known to be precursor of invasive prostate cancer
  - 1–4% of specimens have HGPIN alone (without cancer)
  - Among men found to have HGPIN on initial biopsy, the risk of finding cancer in repeat biopsies results was 22.6%.[15]
  - Men found to have HGPIN on initial biopsy of six cores or less should undergo immediate extended pattern biopsy.
  - When HGPIN is found on initial extended pattern biopsy, close follow up by DRE and PSA measurement is advised.[16]
  - There is no clear consensus as to when repeat biopsy is indicated when HGPIN alone (i.e., no invasive cancer) is found on the initial 12 or more core biopsy.

■ Summary

■ It is important to emphasize that the triggers for biopsy (or rebiopsy) discussed here are not intended as rigid guidelines and that the patient should be assumed to be a candidate for either potentially curative or palliative therapy. The decision to perform a biopsy of the prostate, like all other decisions in medicine, ultimately depends on the judgment of the physician and the overall clinical context.

■ References

1. Balk SP, Ko YJ, Bubley GJ. Biology of prostate-specific antigen. *J Clin Oncol*. 2003;21:383–391.

2. National Comprehensive Cancer Network. Prostate cancer early detection clinical practice guidelines in oncology. *JNCCN*. 2004;2:190–207.

3. Thompson IM, Pauler DK, Goodman PJ, et al. Prevalence of prostate cancer among men with a prostate-specific antigen level ≤ 4.0 ng per milliliter. *N Engl J Med*. 2004;350:2239–2246.

4. Linton KD, Hamdy FC. Early diagnosis and surgical management of prostate cancer. *Cancer Treat Rev*. 2003;29:151–160.

5. Partin AW, Brawer MK, Subong EN, et al. Prospective evaluation of percent free-PSA and complexed-PSA for early detection of prostate cancer. *Prostate Cancer Prostatic Dis*. 1998;1:197–203.

6. Naya Y, Okihara K. Role of complexed PSA in the early detection of prostate cancer. *JNCCN*. 2004;2:209–212.

7. Hessels D, Schalken JA. The use of PCA3 in the diagnosis of prostate cancer. *Nature Revi Urology*. 2009;6(5):255–261.

8. Vickers AJ, Cronin A, Roobal M et al. A four kallikrein panel predicts prstate cancer in men with recent screening:data from the European Randomized Study of Prostate Cancer Screening, Rotterdam. Clinical Cancer Research 2010 April 16 (Epub ahead of print)

9. Patel U. TRUS and prostate biopsy: current status. *Prostate Cancer Prostatic Dis*. 2004;7:208–220.

10. Kampel LJ. Challenging problems in advanced malignancy: Case 2. Disseminated intravascular coagulation in metastatic hormone-refractory prostate cancer. *J Clin Oncol*. 2003;21: 3170–3171.

11. Mian BM. Prostate biopsy strategies: current state of the art. *JNCCN*. 2004;2:213–222.

12. Liu IJ, Macy M, Lai YH, Terris MK. Critical evaluation of the current indications for transitional zone biopsies. *Urology.* 2001;57:1117–1120.

13. Epstein JI. Diagnosis and reporting of limited adenocarcinoma of the prostate on needle biopsy. *Mod Path.* 2004;17:307–315.

14. Evans AJ. Alpha-methylacyl CoA racemase (P504S): overview and potential uses in diagnostic pathology as applied to prostate needle biopsies. *J Clin Pathol.* 2003; 56:892–897.

15. O'Dowd GJ, Miller MC, Orozco R, Veltri RW. Analysis of repeated biopsy results within 1 year after a noncancer diagnosis. *Urology.* 2000;55:553–558.

16. Parsons JK, Partin AW. Clinical interpretation of prostate biopsy reports. *Urology.* 2006;67:452–457.

CHAPTER 3

Pathology of Prostate Cancer

■ Histologic Types

- ■ Adenocarcinoma
  - • 95% of prostate cancers are adenocarcinomas.
    - ■ Acinar adenocarcinoma is the most common.
      - • 75–85% are in the peripheral zone
      - • 10–15% are in the transitional zone or central zone
      - • 10–15% are in the central zone[1]
      - • 85% are multifocal[2]
    - ■ Ductal adenocarcinoma makes up less than 1% of prostatic adenocarcinoma.
      - • More commonly located in periurethral ducts
      - • Histologically similar to endometrial cancer but retains prostate markers
      - • May present in more advanced stage
      - • Confers worse prognosis
    - ■ Mucinous carcinoma and signet ring carcinoma
      - • Very rare
      - • Tend to behave aggressively[3]
  - ■ Less common tumors of the prostate[4]
    - • Neuroendocrine/small cell prostate cancer
      - ■ Arise from Kulchitsky cells in the prostatic basal epithelium
      - ■ May stain positive for
        - • Neuron specific enolase
        - • Chromogranin A (can also be measured in blood)
        - • Synaptophysin
      - ■ Commonly associated with combined Gleason scores of 8–10
      - ■ Possible low PSA level in proportion to the known tumor burden

- Tendency for brief responses to androgen-suppressive therapy
- Tendency to form large, bulky primary prostatic masses
- Visceral (liver, lung, peritoneal, and central nervous system) involvement more common than in lower-grade prostate cancer, in which bone and lymph node pattern predominates
- Can present de novo or on rebiopsy of patients years after initial diagnosis of low- to intermediate-grade adenocarcinoma, particularly in the elderly
- Overall poor prognosis[5] when high-grade neuroendocrine features predominate
- Pure small cell carcinoma may be associated with secretory syndromes similar to small cell lung cancer.[6]
- Small cell cancer generally does not respond to hormone therapy. Platinum-based regimens similar to those used in pulmonary small cell cancer are commonly employed in treatment.
  - Transitional cell carcinoma
    - Secondary invasion of prostate from primary bladder cancer
      - Can be difficult to distinguish from high-grade (poorly differentiated) prostate cancer
    - Primary transitional cell cancer of the prostate arises in the distal prostatic ducts.
- Other malignancies found in the prostate
  - Lymphoma/chronic lymphocytic leukemia
  - Sarcoma
    - Rhabdomyosarcoma in children
    - Leiomyosarcoma
    - Angiosarcoma
      - More commonly a secondary cancer in patients previously radiated for prostate or other pelvic malignancies
  - Metastatic tumors
    - Metastatic solid tumors are rare.
    - Metastases from lung cancer and melanoma have been observed.[7]

■ Tumor Grade (Adenocarcinoma)

- Adenocarcinoma currently graded using the Gleason score[8]
  - Based on glandular architecture, not cytologic grade
  - Recognizes heterogeneity in prostate neoplasms
  - Depends on evaluation of the most prominent pattern and the next most common histological pattern
    - Each of the two patterns is graded on a scale of 1–5 (the more undifferentiated, the higher the score) (**Figures 3-1**, **3-2**, and **3-3**).
    - The combined Gleason score is reported as the sum of the two most common patterns (i.e., Gleason $3+3=6$ or Gleason $4+5=9$; **Table 3-1**).
  - Distribution of Gleason scores depends on type of specimen (**Figure 3-3**).
    - Scores of specimens from transurethral resection of the prostate (TURP) are more commonly 2–4, because tumors in the transition zone are typically low grade.
    - Prostatectomy specimens may be skewed toward lower- and intermediate-grade tumors as a result of case selection.

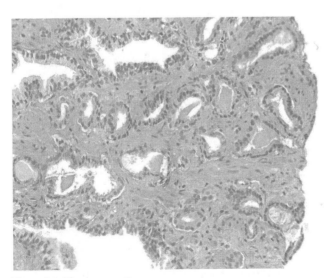

Figure 3-1 Gleason score 3.

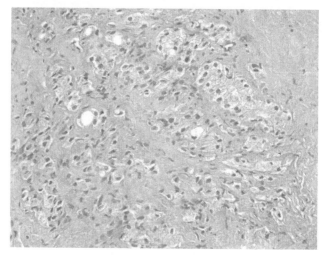

Figure 3-2 Gleason score 4.

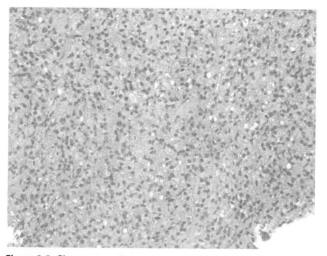

Figure 3-3 Gleason score 5.

- Increasing Gleason score correlates with increased risk of
  - Extraprostatic extension
  - Seminal vesicle involvement
  - Lymph node metastases
  - Positive surgical margins at prostatectomy
  - Worse overall prognosis

Table 3-1 Distribution of Gleason Scores in Prostatectomy Specimens

Gleason Score (sum)[3]	Distribution*	Differentiation
2–4 (low)	6.0%	Well
5–7 (intermediate)	84.3%	Moderate
8–10 (high)	9.7%	Poor

*Refers to distribution of Gleason scores in prostatectomy specimens.

■ Additional Pathologic Findings

- Extent of cancer
  - TRUS-guided biopsies in general do not yield information on the extent of the cancer.
    - On occasion, tissue containing cancer is obtained from the seminal vesicles. Although positive seminal vesicles correlates with distant metastases, artifactual introduction of cancer-containing material may make this finding difficult to interpret.
- Perineural invasion (PNI)
  - The finding of PNI was initially thought to predict for higher pathologic stage, but the preponderance of data suggests that when other pathological findings are controlled for, PNI is not an independent adverse factor.[9]
- Volume of cancer
  - Measures include:
    - Number of positive cores
    - Percentage of each core that is involved by cancer
    - Length of each core (in mm) involved by cancer
  - The usefulness of these measures in predicting final pathologic stage or outcome is not clear at this time.

■ Role of Pathology in Prostate Cancer Risk Assessment

- Although any of the factors discussed can be used to predict pathologic stage and sometimes risk of progression, risk assessment currently depends on combining various factors and comparing them against an existing database. This is discussed in the next chapter.

■ References

1. Carroll PR, Lee KL, Fuks Z, Kantoff PW, et al. Cancer of the prostate. In: DeVita VT, Hellman S, Rosenberg SA, eds. *Cancer: Principles and Practice of Oncology*, 6th ed. Philadelphia: Lippincott, Williams and Wilkins; 2001.

2. Byar DP, Mostofi FK. Carcinoma of the prostate: prognostic evaluation of certain pathologic features in 208 radical prostatectomies. Examined by the step-section technique. *Cancer.* 1972;30:5–13.

3. Epstein JI. Pathology. In: Kantoff P, Carroll PR, D'Amico AV, eds. *Prostate Cancer: Principles and Practice.* Philadelphia: Lippincott, Williams and Wilkins; 2002:232–243.

4. Oh WK, Hurwitz M, Richie JP, D'Amico AV, Kantoff PW, et al. Neoplasms of the prostate. In: Kufe DW, Pollock RE, Weichselbaum RR, et al., eds. *Cancer Medicine.* Hamilton, Ontario: BC Decker; 2003:1707–1740.

5. True L. Why we must better understand neuroendocrine differentiation in prostate cancer (Editorial). *J Urol.* 2004;171:443–444.

6. Sim SJ, Glassman AB, Ro JY, Lee JJ, Logothetis CJ, Liu FJ. Serum calcitonin in small cell carcinoma of the prostate. *Ann Clin Lab Sci.* 1996;26:487–495.

7. Zein TA, Huben R, Lane W, Pontes JE, Englander LS. Secondary tumors of the prostate. *J Urol.* 1985;133:615–616.

8. Gleason DF, Mellinger GT. Prediction of prognosis for prostatic adenocarcinoma by combined histological grading and clinical staging. *J Urol.* 1974;111:58–64.

9. Yossepowitch O, Trabulsi EJ, Kattan MW, Scardino PT. Predictive factors in prostate cancer: implications for decision making. *Cancer Invest.* 2003;21:465–480.

Section III
Clinical State: Localized Disease

CHAPTER 4

Staging and Risk Assessment

■ Introduction

Prostate cancers are a heterogeneous mix of neoplasms with varying and often unpredictable clinical behaviors. Many of the cancers detected by PSA determination may never cause symptoms or threaten the lives of the men harboring them. The challenge, to quote Dr. Willard Whitmore, is to determine if "...cure is possible for men in whom it is necessary, and is cure necessary for men in whom it is possible."

▨ Staging and risk assessment prior to definitive or potentially curative therapy depend on accurate assessment of the following:

- Overall health status of the patient
  - ▨ Comorbidities that might impact type of treatment
  - ▨ Estimated life expectancy
- Local extent of the disease
  - ▨ Extent of tumor and location within the prostate
  - ▨ Extracapsular extension
  - ▨ Seminal vesicle, bladder, or rectal involvement
- Presence or absence of metastatic disease
  - ▨ Regional lymph node involvement
  - ▨ Distant lymph node involvement
  - ▨ Skeletal metastases
  - ▨ Visceral metastases
- Factors intrinsic to the patient's tumor
  - ▨ Histologic grade
  - ▨ PSA
  - ▨ Other markers, such as PCA3, TMPRSS2–ERG fusion product

This chapter first reviews appropriate staging techniques for the primary tumor (T), nodes (N), and metastatic disease (M). For patients whose disease remains localized, and thus potentially curable, the integration of anatomic staging with other biologic factors is discussed with a view toward risk assessment, which is critical in choosing the appropriate therapy.

■ Staging

The TNM Staging System for Prostate Cancer

- ▓ The TNM stage defines the local extent of disease as well as the presence or absence of regional and distant spread of the cancer.
- ▓ The TNM system of staging prostate cancer is purely anatomic; it does not include:
  - ◦ Tumor grade
  - ◦ PSA levels or other biomarkers
- ▓ Initial TNM staging is clinical
  - ◦ Based on the DRE alone
- ▓ Pathologic TNM refers to prostatectomy findings.
- ▓ This book uses the 2002 version of the TNM system (see **Figure 4-1**)[1].

Determining Local Extent of Disease (T Stage)

- ▓ DRE
  - ◦ By definition, T1 tumors are not clinically detectable by DRE.
    - ▓ If a cancer is found incidental to a TURP performed for BPH, it is staged T1a or T1b, depending on the percentage of the tissue that contains cancer.
    - ▓ If a cancer is found in the result of a biopsy done because of an elevated PSA level alone, it is staged T1c.
    - ▓ Tumors that are clearly palpable are staged T2, and those that extend beyond the prostate are staged either T3 or T4.
  - ◦ DRE is somewhat subjective and operator dependent but still provides useful information for determining the T stage in the TNM system.

TUMOR STAGE

T0 No evidence of primary tumor

T1 Nondetectable by PE or imaging
  T1a Incidental finding at TURP ≤ 5% of tissue involved
  T1b Incidental finding at TURP > 5% of tissue involved
  T1c Tumor found at biopsy triggered by PSA only

T2 Tumor detectable by PE or imaging
  T2a Tumor involves ≤ ½ of one lobe
  T2b Tumor involves > ½ of one lobe
  T2c Tumor involves both lobes

T3 Tumor extends beyond capsule
  T3a Unilateral or bilateral extracapsular extension
  T3b Tumor involves one or both seminal vesicles

T4 Tumor is fixed or invades adjacent structures
  T4a Involvement of bladder neck, external sphincter, or rectum
  T4b Involvement of levator muscles or tumor fixed to pelvic sidewalls

NODAL STAGING (N)

Nx Nodal status is not assessed
N0 No evidence of nodal metastases
N1 Regional nodes involved

STAGING OF METASTATIC DISEASE (M)

Mx Metastatic disease not assessed
M0 No evidence of metastatic disease
M1 Metastatic disease in nonregional nodes and other sites

Figure 4-1 TNM staging of prostate cancer.

* The distinction between T1 (nonpalpable) and T2 (palpable) disease may not always be straightforward. A clearly negative DRE or one that reveals an unequivocal nodule or mass is not always the case.

- How to stage vague areas of induration or differences in consistency in different parts of the prostate is unclear.
  - Because of the subjectivity of the DRE, it would be prudent to be very conservative in assigning a clinical T stage by DRE because overstaging could result in denying the patient potentially curative therapy.
  - Similarly, it can be difficult to distinguish organ-confined cancer from extraprostatic spread in the absence of a grossly abnormal DRE.
- Because clinical staging of the primary tumor is so subjective, it is not surprising that understaging has been reported to be as high as 30–60%.[2,3] Thus, a variety of imaging techniques have been used to improve the accuracy of T staging. Although these techniques may be useful adjuncts, the clinical T stage is based only on DRE.
- Imaging
  - TRUS and computed tomography (CT)
    - Generally not sufficiently sensitive to be useful in distinguishing among early T stages.[4]
    - CT can demonstrate large or bulky disease or bladder involvement, when extensive, and may be useful in evaluating the abdomen and pelvis for metastatic disease in high-risk patients (see page 51).
  - Magnetic resonance imaging (MRI) with surface or endorectal coil
    - Usefulness in patients with clinically T1 tumors not established (tumors may be too small to evaluate by MRI)
    - When visualized, prostate cancers appear hypodense on T2 images.
    - Presence of intact capsule or even smooth capsular bulge supports diagnosis of organ-confined (T2) disease.
    - MRI useful in diagnosing
      - Extracapsular spread (T3a)
        - Specificity is high (95%)
        - Sensitivity is no more than 50%[5]
      - Seminal vesicle involvement (T3b)[6]
    - MRI also provides information about status of nearby nodes and bony structures

- Magnetic resonance spectroscopy (MRS)
  - MRS is an experimental technique in which spectroscopic data are acquired at the same time the MRI is done.
  - Normal prostate tissue is high in citrate, while areas of prostate cancer are rich in choline.
  - MR images and spectroscopic data can be superimposed to enhance visualization of abnormal areas. See **Figure 4-2**.

Determining Nodal Status (N Stage)

The accurate assessment of nodal status in patients with early prostate cancer remains a challenge for clinicians. Imaging techniques currently in use are increasingly able to detect very minor lymph node enlargement. When faced with an equivocally positive imaging result, and particularly when the patient's other risk factors make metastatic disease unlikely, the burden is on the clinician to prove that the abnormal node indeed contains cancer and, if so, that it is prostate cancer rather than a second malignancy, such as lymphoma.

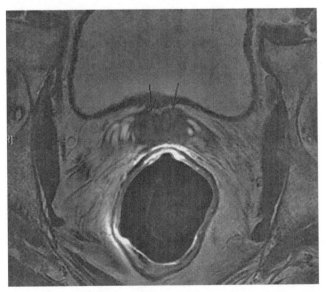

Figure 4-2 Prostatic MR showing seminal vesicle invasion by prostate cancer.

- Imaging techniques
  - CT
    - True positives are rare when the PSA level is less than 10 ng/ml, unless the patient has high-grade cancer.
    - Nodes larger than 1 cm are considered suspicious.
    - Sensitivity is 30–78%.
    - Specificity is 77–97%.[7]
  - Abdominal pelvic MRI
    - Sensitivity and specificity similar to CT but more expensive
    - May be useful in patients who cannot tolerate intravenous (IV) contrast dye
  - Radioimmunoscintigraphy—radiolabeled indium In 111 capromab pendetide (ProstaScint®)
    - Uses a radiolabeled murine monoclonal immunoglobulin G antibody against an intracellular epitope of prostatic-specific membrane antigen
    - Requires imaging at 30 minutes to 120 hours after injection
    - Usefulness in early prostate cancer not established
    - May be more useful in patients with rising PSA levels after primary therapy
  - Positron emission tomography (PET)
    - Possibly useful in evaluating nodal and visceral metastases
    - Less sensitive than bone scanning for detection of bone metastases
    - Not useful in distinguishing benign from malignant process in the prostate itself
    - Replacement of glucose label by testosterone may increase sensitivity/specificity.
    - At this time, PET is not approved for reimbursement when used for prostate cancer.
  - Superparamagnetic nanoparticles with high-resolution MRI
    - Highly lymphotropic marker
    - In an initial report, all of 63 nodes (from 33 patients) that were positive at surgery were identified preoperatively by this technique.

- 41 of the 63 (71%) were negative by preoperative MRI.[8]
- This procedure is still considered experimental and awaits validation.
- Biopsy
  - Performing a biopsy of suspicious lymph nodes should be strongly considered before therapy with curative intent is abandoned when:
    - Nodes are borderline in size.
    - The clinical suspicion for metastatic disease is low.
    - Pattern of abnormal lymph node is unusual.
      - Prostate cancer typically involves obturator, iliac, and para-aortic nodes.
      - Enlargement of mesenteric nodes only should raise suspicion for lymphoma.
    - Biopsies of most nodes can now be performed by image-guided techniques.

Determining Metastatic Disease Status (M Stage)

Prostate adenocarcinoma typically spreads to bone and lymph nodes. Late in the disease course, and particularly in patients with high-grade, neuroendocrine, or small cell varieties, visceral metastases can be seen involving the mesentery, gastrointestinal (GI) tract, liver, lungs, and skin. Parenchymal brain metastases are rare, but direct extension from dural or skull metastases is common.

- Imaging osseous structures
  - Routine x-ray studies
    - Metastases appear blastic in most cases.
    - Insufficiently sensitive to detect early bone metastases
      - In order for bone metastases to be detected by plain radiographs, there must be at least a 50% change in the bone density.[7]
  - Radionuclide bone scintigraphy (bone scan) (see **Figure 4-3**)
    - Very sensitive technique for diagnosing bone metastases using technetium Tc 99
      - Shortage of Tc 99 has led to the introduction of other isotopes

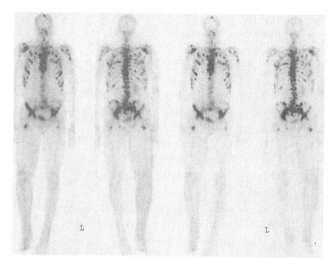

Figure 4-3 Radionuclide Tc 99 bone scan showing extensive osseous metastases from prostate cancer.

- Isotope preferentially taken up at sites of bone metastases, allowing determination of the location and number of skeletal metastases and the intensity of uptake at each site
- Low yield (~1%) in patients with:
  - PSA level of less than 10 ng/ml
  - Combined Gleason score of less than 7
  - T stage lower than T3[9]
- Remaining Tc 99 not taken up by osseous structures circulates in blood and is excreted by the kidneys, resulting in nephrogram effect when renal function is normal
  - Unilateral or bilateral hydronephrosis may be incidental finding on bone scan
  - Superscan
    - In patients with extensive skeletal involvement, all the isotope can be taken up by metastatic sites, leaving insufficient concentrations in the blood to allow visualization of the kidneys, ureters, and bladder, despite normal renal function. These scans are referred to as "superscans."

- It is important to be aware of this, because in some cases, the abnormal uptake in bone is so diffuse that no single area appears "hotter" than any other. In this situation, the absence of renal visualization (again assuming normal renal function) may be the only clue that the scan is indeed abnormal.
- False-positives and confounding factors
  - Trauma
  - Degenerative joint disease
  - Prior surgery
  - Paget's disease
  - Bone islands, infarcts, hemangiomas, and fibrous dysplasia
- Paradoxical flare during therapy
  - Bone repair in response to anticancer treatment (most often androgen deprivation) may result in a temporary increase in the intensity of abnormal uptake at known metastatic sites. This must be distinguished from true progression of disease when the bone scan is used to monitor treatment response.
- In many cases, experienced clinicians, in conjunction with imaging experts, can make the distinction between benign abnormalities and true positives.
  - When questions remain, further imaging by either CT with bone windows and/or MRI may be helpful.
  - If the issue remains unresolved, biopsy may be necessary.
  - As always, the decision to perform a biopsy is a judgment based on the overall clinical scenario. For example, if the patient is not a candidate for curative therapy, the issue becomes moot. On the other hand, if the patient is a candidate for a curative approach and the clinical features (T stage, PSA, and Gleason score) are all favorable, the threshold for triggering biopsy consideration should be low.

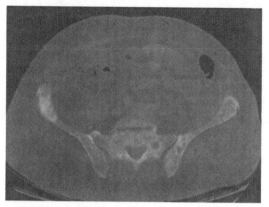

Figure 4-4 CT of the pelvis showing extensive blastic metastases.

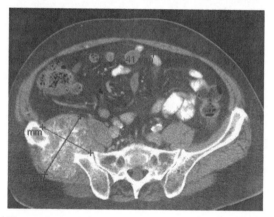

Figure 4-5 Atypical expansile and destructive bone metastasis in patient whose prostate cancer had squamous features.

- Imaging for nonosseous metastases
  - CT
    - Commonly used to detect nodal or visceral metastases
    - Low yield in patients with PSA level of less than 10 ng/ml who have less than T3 disease and combined Gleason score of less than 7[10]
    - Ability of CT to detect small nodes may increase sensitivity but decrease specificity

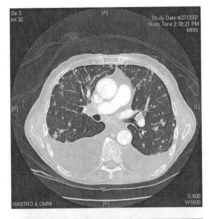

Figure 4-6
Lung metastases
and pleural effusion
secondary to prostate
cancer.

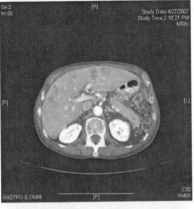

Figure 4-7
Liver metastases in a
patient with prostate
cancer.

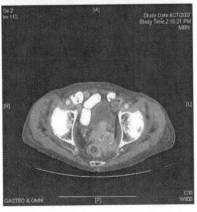

Figure 4-8
Large recurrent prostate
cancer between rectum
and bladder.

- MRI
  - More expensive than CT
  - Sensitivity and selectivity about the same
  - May be useful in high-risk patients who cannot tolerate IV contrast dye needed for CT
- Radioimmunoscintigraphy
  - See within Determining Nodal Status (N Stage), page 53
- PET
  - Also see within Determining Nodal Status (N Stage), page 53
  - The use of other metabolites in PET (fDHT) scanning for prostate cancer is currently under investigation.
- Performing a biopsy of suspicious lesions should be considered if the patient's disease is otherwise potentially curable, particularly if the clinical features make the likelihood of metastases low.

Summary Recommendations for Imaging in Newly Diagnosed Prostate Cancer

- Patients with favorable-risk prostate cancer (PSA < 10 ng/ml, Gleason score < 7, and primary tumor < T3) who are asymptomatic do not require imaging to rule out metastatic disease.
- Patients who have symptoms suggestive of metastases should undergo appropriate imaging no matter what the PSA level, Gleason score, or T stage.
- MRI with endorectal coil is useful in determining the local extent of disease, particularly in patients with clinical stage (by DRE) of T2 or higher.
- Higher-risk patients should undergo radionuclide bone scanning and CT scanning of the abdomen and pelvis.
- Bone windows should be included whenever CT scans are conducted.
- The value of all the imaging techniques discussed earlier is highly dependent on the experience and skill of those performing and interpreting the studies. The usefulness of the studies may vary from center to center. In choosing the staging workup, it is important that the clinician is

knowledgeable about the capabilities, strengths, and weaknesses of the imaging team being used.

■ It remains axiomatic that when imaging suggests distant metastases, the burden is on the clinician to prove that the patient has incurable metastatic disease. Whenever the imaging results are discordant with the clinical scenario, further workup that includes additional imaging, and possibly biopsy, should be strongly considered before relegating the disease to an incurable status. To paraphrase a famous legal mind, "If the clinical picture doesn't fit, you must acquit!"

■ Having said that, in some cases it may be impossible to prove whether or not an abnormal area on a bone scan or CT scan represents a metastasis or a benign process.

　• In these cases, a pragmatic decision must be made.

　　■ If the patient is otherwise fit and the overall prognostic features are favorable, it is not unreasonable to offer potentially curative therapy, as long as the patient and his family understand that the lesion in question may ultimately declare itself.

　　■ On the other hand, in patients with unfavorable risk profiles in whom the index of suspicion is high, it is also reasonable to start androgen deprivation therapy, with a view toward definitive therapy in the future if the lesion either remains stable or regresses and no new lesions develop.

■ Risk Assessment

■ Despite careful evaluation of the T stage and thorough imaging to exclude metastatic disease, many men who undergo curative therapy experience relapse or are found at surgery to have more extensive local disease than expected.

　• For those patients, primary therapy with radiation or surgery is not likely to be curative. If these patients could be identified prior to definitive local therapy, they could be spared surgery or radiation or they could be offered neoadjuvant therapy to reduce the risk of treatment failure. Validated tools for risk categorization are also important for the development of clinical trials.

- The following individual factors have been identified as correlating with a more advanced stage and poor outcome:
  - Increasing PSA, percent free PSA, and PSA velocity[11]
  - PCA3 score
  - Increasing clinical stage by DRE
  - Increasing Gleason score
  - Increasing cancer volume as indicated by percentage of cores or number of cores involved
  - Race
    - Worse prognosis in African American and Caribbean men
  - Increasing age
  - Increasing molecular markers
    - IL-6
    - TGFβ
- Combined risk assessments
  - Although any of the individual markers or studies listed earlier may be useful in predicting final pathologic stage, risk of relapse, and maybe even survival, combining factors has been shown to be more accurate.[12]
  - The three most important factors are
    - PSA
    - T stage by DRE
    - Combined Gleason score
- A quick glance at **Table 4-1** should reveal the limitations of such a simple grouping. Patients often have a mix of favorable and unfavorable factors. Also, this table does not distinguish the patient with a PSA level of 10 ng/ml from one with a level of 2 ng/ml, or the patient with a Gleason score of 10 from one with a Gleason score of 8.
- Nomograms and tables for risk assessment
  - Modern risk assessment is based on the use of multiple variables applied in a continuous fashion, as exemplified by various tables and nomograms. These tables and nomograms employ a number of pretreatment factors to predict either pathologic stage at surgery or freedom from progression based on a preexisting database. The two most common tools used are the Partin tables and the Kattan nomogram.

Table 4-1 Risk Assessment Based on PSA, Gleason Score, and T Stage[13]

Risk Level	PSA (ng/mL)	Gleason Score	T Stage
Good	≤ 10	≤ 6	≤ T2a
Intermediate	10–20	7	T2b
High	> 20	8, 9, or 10	≥ T3

Data from D'Amico A. Combined modality staging in predicting prostate specific antigen outcome after definitive local therapy for men with clinically localized prostate cancer. In: Kantoff P, Carrol PR, D'Amico AV, *eds. Prostate Cancer: Principles and Practice. Philadelphia: Lippincott, Williams and Wilkins; 2002:254–268.*

- The Partin tables[14]
  - The Partin tables predict pathologic stage at surgery using
    - Serum PSA level
    - Gleason score
    - T stage by DRE
  - The original Partin tables are widely available. However, they are somewhat cumbersome, as each prediction requires reference to a different set of tables. Moreover, their utility in predicting prognosis and outcome is limited, because they use discrete cut-off values. A new computerized version that incorporates additional risk factors can be found at the following Web site: http://urology.jhu.edu/prostate/partintables.php.
- The Kattan nomogram[15]
  - This nomogram can be used online at http://www.mskcc.org/mskcc/html/10088.cfm and can be downloaded.
  - It appears superior to tables in predicting outcomes.[16]
  - The Kattan nomogram prompts the user to enter the following
    - Pretreatment PSA level
    - Primary Gleason score
    - Secondary Gleason score
    - Clinical T stage

- Radiotherapy dose
- Preoperative IL-6 level (optional)
- Preoperative TGFβ level (optional)
- Whether or not neoadjuvant hormone therapy is to be given
- More recent versions prompt for information about the extent of cancer in the biopsy cores.
- The program returns the:
  - Pathologic stage probability if the patient is to have radical prostatectomy
  - 5-year progression-free probability for
    - Radical prostatectomy
    - External-beam radiotherapy (EBRT) with or without neoadjuvant hormone therapy
    - Brachytherapy with or without neoadjuvant hormone therapy
- Newer versions of the program contain a number of other utilities that are useful for clinicians dealing with prostate cancer.
- The two major advantages of the Kattan nomogram are:
  - Predictions are based on exact PSA values and Gleason scores rather than ranges.
  - Primary and secondary Gleason scores are entered separately rather than as a sum.

Note: Not all the end points in either of the two predictive models are equally well validated. Although they are useful tools, these calculations should not be used alone in determining treatment decisions.

■ References

1. Hull GW, Rabbani F, Abbas F, Wheeler TM, Kattan MW, Scardino PT. Cancer control with radical prostatectomy alone in 1,000 consecutive patients. *J Urol.* 2002;167(Pt 1):528–534.
2. D'Amico A, Whittington R, Schnall M, et al. The impact of the inclusion of endorectal coil magnetic resonance imaging in a multivariate analysis to predict clinically unsuspected extraprostatic cancer. *Cancer.* 1995;75:2368–2372.

3. Mukamel E, Hanna J, deKernion JB. Pitfalls in preoperative staging in prostate cancer. *Urology.* 1987;30:318–321.

4. Engeler CE, Wasserman NF, Zhang G. Preoperative assessment of prostatic carcinoma by computerized tomography. Weaknesses and new perspectives. *Urology.* 1992;40:346–350.

5. Yu KK, Hricak H, Alagappan R, Chernoff DM, Bacchetti P, Zaloudek CJ. Detection of extracapsular extension of prostate carcinoma with endorectal and phased-array coil MR imaging: multivariate feature analysis. *Radiology.* 1997;202:697–702.

6. Bezzi M, Kressel HY, Allen KS, et al. Prostatic carcinoma: staging with MR imaging at 1.5 T. *Radiology.* 1988;169:339–346.

7. Wefer AE, Hricak H. Imaging and staging of prostate cancer. In: Kantoff P, Carroll PR, D'Amico AV, eds. *Prostate Cancer: Principles and Practice.* Philadelphia: Lippincott, Williams and Wilkins; 2002:269–286.

8. Harisinghani MG, Barentsz J, Hahn PF, et al. Noninvasive detection of clinically occult lymph-node metastases in prostate cancer. *N Engl J Med.* 2003;348:2491–2499.

9. Gleave ME, Coupland D, Drachenberg D, et al. Ability of serum prostate-specific antigen to predict normal bone scans in patients with newly diagnosed prostate cancer. *Urology.* 1996;47:708–712.

10. Huncharek M, Muscat J. Serum prostatic-specific antigen as a predictor of staging abdominal/pelvic computed tomography in newly diagnosed prostate cancer. *Abdom Imaging.* 1996;21:364–367.

11. D'Amico AV, Chen MH, Roehl KA, Catalona WJ. Preoperative PSA velocity and the risk of death from prostate cancer after radical prostatectomy. *N Engl J Med.* 2004;351:125–135.

12. Partin AW, Kattan MW, Subong EN, et al. Combination of prostate-specific antigen, clinical stage, and Gleason score to predict pathological stage of localized prostate cancer. A multi-institutional update. *JAMA.* 1997;277:1445–1451.

13. D'Amico A. Combined modality staging in predicting prostate-specific antigen outcome after definitive local therapy for men with clinically localized prostate cancer. In: Kantoff P, Carroll PR, D'Amico AV, eds. *Prostate Cancer: Principles and Practice.* Philadelphia: Lippincott, Williams and Wilkins; 2002:254–268.

14. Partin AW, Yoo J, Carter HB, et al. The use of prostate specific antigen, clinical stage and Gleason score to predict pathologic stage in men with localized prostate cancer. *J Urol.* 1993;150:110–114.

15. Kattan MW, Eastham JA, Stapleton AM, Wheeler TM, Scardino PT. A preoperative nomogram for disease recurrence following radical prostatectomy for prostate cancer. *J Natl Cancer Inst.* 1998;90:766–771.

16. Scher H, Leibel SA, Fuks Z, Cordon-Cardo C, Scardino P, et al. Cancer of the prostate. In: DeVita VT, Hellman S, Rosenberg SA, eds. *Cancer: Principles and Practice of Oncology.* 7th ed. Philadelphia: Lippincott, Williams and Wilkins; 2005:1192–1259.

CHAPTER 5

Primary Management of Favorable- and Intermediate-Risk Prostate Cancer

■ Introduction

▪ Men with newly diagnosed and clinically localized prostate cancer face a bewildering and frequently anxiety-provoking array of choices. Lacking certainty that any individual therapy or combination/permutation thereof is better than any other, the clinicians caring for them may fare no better. This chapter reviews the various options for the management of clinically localized prostate cancer as well as their advantages and disadvantages and their efficacy in achieving long-term control of the disease.

▪ *It should be emphasized and made abundantly clear to all patients presenting with localized prostate cancer that there is absolutely no certainty that one treatment modality (or combination) is superior to any other.* The lack of randomized trials, the variation in end points, and the ongoing evolution of surgical (standard open retropubic prostatectomy → laparoscopic prostatectomy → robotic prostatectomy) as well as external-beam radiotherapy (2-dimensional nonconformal radiation → 3-dimensional conformal radiation → intensity-modulated radiation → image-guided radiotherapy) and brachytherapy techniques result in constantly shifting targets that make comparison difficult. At the same time, it is clear that, for some subsets of patients, enough data exists such that options can be narrowed.

■ The Initial Management Consultation

■ Once the diagnosis of prostate cancer has been established, a decision must be made about the best treatment for each individual patient.

■ The patient will certainly want to discuss options with his urologist and primary physician.
- He may also be offered consultation with a radiation oncologist.
- Medical oncologists are increasingly involved in primary treatment decisions for patients with high-risk disease and for those who seek an "unbiased" opinion about managing even favorable lesions.

■ These consultations are critical for the patient, because the choice of therapy is bound to be life altering.

■ Sufficient time for a full discussion of all options should be allowed.

■ For each modality, the risks and benefits should be reviewed in detail. The likelihood of cure as well as the possible impact on bowel, urinary, and sexual function should be explained.

■ The physician should attempt to learn as much as possible about the patient, his individual needs, and unique concerns.

■ Although family members, friends, and significant others are often present during the visit, the patient should be given the opportunity to discuss sexual and other personal issues privately.

■ Management options for clinically localized prostate cancer are shown in **Table 5-1**.

■ Surgery for Clinically Localized Prostate Cancer
Radical Retropubic Prostatectomy

■ Nerve-sparing or anatomic radical retropubic prostatectomy is the most common surgical procedure for prostate cancer.
- Majority now done using robotically assisted techniques.

■ Involves resection of the prostate, seminal vesicles, and vas deferens

Table 5-1 Management Options for Localized Prostate Cancer

POTENTIALLY CURATIVE APPROACHES

- Surgical
  - Radical retropubic prostatectomy
  - Laparoscopic radical prostatectomy
  - Robotic laparascopic prostatectomy
  - Transperineal prostatectomy
- Radiotherapy (with or without hormone therapy)
  - EBRT
    - 3DCRT
    - IMRT\IGRT
  - Brachytherapy
    - Iodine I125
    - Palladium Pd103
    - Iridium Ir192 high-dose rate
  - EBRT plus brachytherapy
  - Hypofractionated radiotherapy

NONCURATIVE APPROACHES

- Hormone therapy
- Watchful waiting or active surveillance

- Generally involves lymphadenectomy for the removal of pelvic lymph nodes
  - The need for lymphadenectomy in low-risk patients is not clear.
  - Lymphadenectomy should be considered for higher-risk patients[1]:
    - Clinical stage of T2 or higher
    - PSA level of greater than 10 ng/ml
    - Gleason score of greater than 6
    - Extensive cancer involvement of biopsy cores
    - ~1% chance of node involvement in lower-risk patients
  - Ultimately, the decision regarding lymphadenectomy is a surgical judgment. The nomogram discussed in Chapter 4 may be useful in the selection of patients for pelvic lymph node dissection (J. Eastham, MD, oral communication, 3/06).

■ Advantages of radical retropubic prostatectomy
  * Standard operation with long record of excellent cancer control (see Outcomes with Radical Retropubic Prostatectomy).
  * Local cancer completely removed
  * Symptoms due to concurrent BPH relieved
  * Accurate pathologic staging obtained, allowing determination of need for adjuvant therapy (see Chapter 6)
  * Psychological advantage of knowing the cancer has been removed
  * Avoids protracted course of external-beam radiotherapy (EBRT)
  * Risk profile more acceptable to some men compared with external-beam radiotherapy, brachytherapy, and other modalities
  * Avoids the risk of radiation induced second cancers
  * Less bowel toxicity
  * Less risk of chronic obstructive symptoms
■ Outcomes with radical retropubic prostatectomy
  * Excellent record of cancer control, particularly for low-risk patients
    ■ Actuarial nonprogression rates in a number of large series[2–5] (not risk adjusted):
      ■ 5 years: 75–85%
      ■ 10 years: 70–75%
      ■ 15 years: 65–70%
    ■ The series of 1,000 patients with clinically localized prostate cancer (< T3) reported in 2002[2] was recently updated to include 1,716 patients,[6] with a mean follow-up of 6.3 years (range, 1–20 years).
      * Of note, only 7% of the patients died of prostate cancer and only 15% had relapses.
      * **Figure 5-1** shows actuarial biochemical progression-free probability (bPFP) for the entire group.
    ■ PFP depends on
      * Clinical stage (**Figure 5-2**)
      * Gleason score (**Figure 5-3**)
      * Preoperative PSA level (**Figure 5-4**)

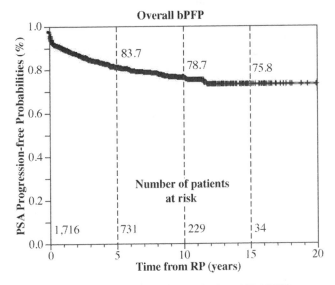

Figure 5-1 Overall bPFP. Courtesy of James Eastham, MD; MSKCC, Medical Graphics; and Fernando Bianco, MD.

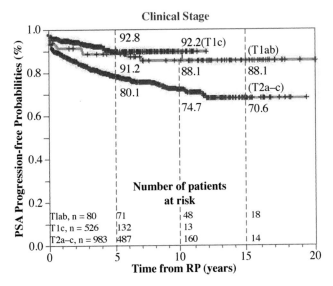

Figure 5-2 bPFP by clinical stage. Courtesy of James Eastham, MD; MSKCC, Medical Graphics; and Fernando Bianco, MD.

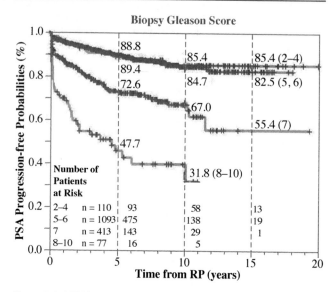

Figure 5-3 bPFP by Gleason score at initial biopsy. Courtesy of James Eastham, MD; MSKCC, Medical Graphics; and Fernando Bianco, MD.

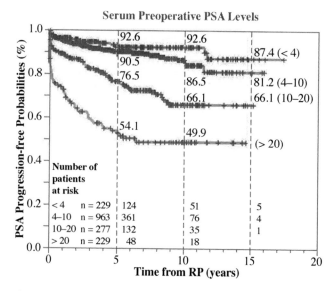

Figure 5-4 bPFP by preoperative PSA level. Courtesy of James Eastham, MD; MSKCC, Medical Graphics; and Fernando Bianco, MD.

- Combined risk stratification (**Figure 5-5**)
    - Low risk
        - T2a or lower, combined Gleason score of 6 or less, and PSA level less than 10 ng/ml
    - Intermediate risk
        - T2b or combined Gleason scores of 7 or PSA level greater than 10 but less than or equal to 20 ng/ml
    - High risk
        - T2c or Gleason score of 8–10 or PSA level of greater than 20 ng/ml
- Pathologic stage[6,7]
    - Postoperative TN (p TN) stage (**Figure 5-6**)
    - Extracapsular extension (**Figure 5-7**)
    - Positive surgical margins (**Figure 5-8**)
- Prostate cancer–specific mortality (PCSM) was evaluated for a cohort of 12,677 patients who underwent radical prostatectomy between 1987 and 2005 at two academic centers.
    - 15-year PCSM was 12% (overall mortality was 38%).
    - PCSM ranged from 5% for good-risk patients to 38% for high-risk patients based on their predictive nomogram.[8]

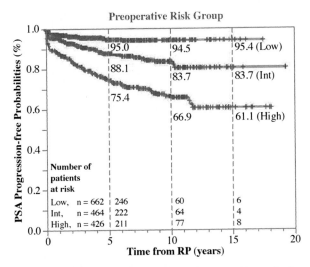

Figure 5-5 bPFP by preoperative risk group. Courtesy of James Eastham, MD; MSKCC, Medical Graphics; and Fernando Bianco, MD.

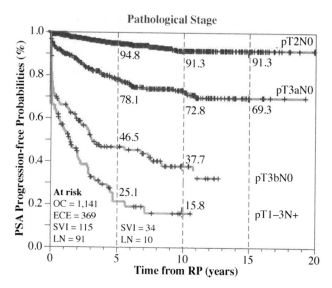

Figure 5-6 bPFP by tumor and node status. ECE = extracapsular extension; LN = lymph node; OC = organ-confined; SVI = seminal vesicle invasion. Courtesy of James Eastham, MD; MSKCC, Medical Graphics; and Fernando Bianco, MD.

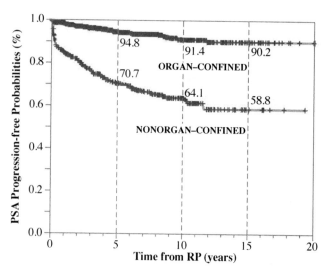

Figure 5-7 bPFP by organ-confined vs. non-organ-confined disease. Courtesy of James Eastham, MD; MSKCC, Medical Graphics; and Fernando Bianco, MD.

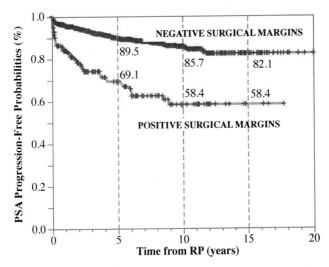

Figure 5-8 bPFP by positive vs. negative surgical margins. Courtesy of James Eastham, MD; MSKCC, Medical Graphics; and Fernando Bianco, MD.

- The data shown above reveal a very good outlook for patients with low-risk disease and even for some with high-risk disease. Clearly, better treatment options are needed for those with higher-risk disease, such as patients with very undifferentiated tumors (Gleason 8–10), advanced local disease (T3b or N1), or very high PSA level at presentation.
- Complications and disadvantages of radical retropubic prostatectomy
  - Short-term complications
    - Radical retropubic prostatectomy is a major surgical procedure.
    - Patients anticipating this operation should undergo general medical evaluation prior to surgery and expect at least several weeks of recovery before full activity is resumed.
    - The procedure requires an inpatient stay of 2–4 days.
  - Perioperative mortality rate (death within 30 days of surgery) of 0.1[9,10]

- Intraoperative complications[11–13]
  - Bleeding
    - Average blood loss of 800–1,000 cc
      - As experience with the procedure grows, average blood loss is decreasing.
    - The use of erythropoietin therapy and autologous donation has reduced the need for allo-transfusion to 2–10%.
  - Rectal tear risk of 0.5%
    - Usually repaired intraoperatively, need for colostomy is rare
  - Obturator nerve injury is rare.
  - Occipital blindness or hearing loss due to hypo-perfusion is extremely rare.
- Postoperative complications[9]
  - Myocardial infarction: 0.4–0.6%
  - Thromboembolic events: 1–1.5%
  - Stricture: 0.5–9%
  - Postoperative bleeding: 0.5%
  - All patients require a temporary indwelling urinary catheter after surgery. Typically, the catheter is removed 7–14 days after surgery.
- Long-term complications
  - The major concerns for most men considering radical prostatectomy are urinary incontinence and impotence.
    - The incidence of sexual complications reported in the literature is extremely variable and, to a large extent, dependent on how they are defined and how aggressively data are collected.
  - Infertility
    - Men anticipating radical prostatectomy (or radiotherapy) should consider sperm banking if they wish to have more children.
  - Anastamotic stricture
    - 0.5–9% in various reports[14]
    - May require urethral dilatation or urethrotomy

- Permanent Incontinence
  - Overall, the risk of permanent incontinence is less than 10% in surgical series.
    - Of these 10%, most report only mild stress incontinence.
    - Less than 5% require pads.
    - 1–2% require surgical procedures to improve urinary control.[1]
    - Risk factors
      - Age older than 70
      - Size of tumor/prostate.
      - Experience of the surgeon.[15]
  - Urinary control may improve slowly over a 12–24-month period.
  - Despite the relatively low incidence of incontinence reported in surgical series, quality of life studies suggest a greater impact. In the Prostate Cancer Outcomes Study (PCOS), which looked at quality of life 5 years after prostatectomy, approximately 15% of patients reported leakage at least two times per day, and approximately 28% wore at least one pad per day.[16] Bowel urgency was also reported by 20% of men in this study.
- Erectile dysfunction
  - Overall erectile dysfunction rates reported in the literature of 40–70%
  - Among 1,870 patients reported by Catalona[15]:
    - 68% retained potency with bilateral nerve sparing
    - 47% remained potent with unilateral nerve sparing
  - Increased risk of impotence with higher T stage tumor
  - Size (of surgical experience) matters
    - Increased risk of impotence when surgeon has performed less than 500 procedures compared with surgeons who have performed more than 1,000 procedures

■ The older the patient, the higher the risk of erectile dysfunction, even with nerve sparing.

Table 5-2 Risk of Postoperative Impotence as a Function of Patient Age

Age (years)	Risk of Impotence (%)[13]
< 50	10
50–59	20
60–69	40
> 70	53

■ Nerve sparing seems to be more effective in younger patients compared with older ones.

■ Preexisting erectile dysfunction and certain comorbidities or medications also increase the risk of erectile dysfunction.

■ For younger, healthy men with no antecedent erectile dysfunction and small tumors, the risk of erectile dysfunction is probably in the 30–40% range. Many men who are sexually active after prostatectomy do require pharmacological assistance (personal communication with James Eastham).

■ Reducing the risk of erectile dysfunction after radical prostatectomy
  * Early use of phosphodiesterase-5 inhibitors
  * Men undergoing radical prostatectomy should understand that return of erectile function may take up to 12–36 months.
* Dry orgasm due to absence of ejaculate
* Climacturia: the passage of small amounts of urine at climax
* Decrease in penile length
* Who should be considered for radical retropubic prostatectomy?
  ■ Patients who in general are candidates for potentially curative therapy with
    * Life expectancy of 10 years or more
    * No serious fixed comorbidity
    * Clinically localized disease and low to intermediate risk factors as described earlier

■ The data shown in Figures 5.1–5.8 indicate that even some patients with advanced locoregional disease or other unfavorable prognostic factors do well with prostatectomy. These patients should be made aware of the higher risk of failure and also be offered radiotherapy. Where available, they also can be offered participation in neoadjuvant clinical trials.

  * Surgery is generally not recommended if there is compelling evidence of nodal involvement.

■ Younger patients

  * Whitmore's rule (paraphrased)—*Never operate on any man over the age of 70 unless his father walks in the door with him.*

  * Surgery should not be ruled out based on age alone.

  * Patients older than 70 years (usually in their early 70s) who are physiologically fit can be considered for surgery.

  * The availability of other potentially curative options should be strongly kept in mind when considering surgery for older patients or young patients with fixed comorbidities that increase surgical risk.

■ Patients with potentially curable disease who cannot undergo radiotherapy (see EBRT on page 83)

* As discussed earlier, no single factor other than the presence of metastatic disease or a technically inoperable tumor should rule out prostatectomy as a potentially curative option.

  ■ The use of nomograms in assessing therapy options for localized prostate cancer is becoming more common.

    * Nomograms allow the inclusion of multiple factors, most commonly pretreatment PSA level, clinical stage, and Gleason score, in order to predict posttherapy outcomes.

    * As data mature, newer factors, such as serum IL-6, TGFβ, and human kallikrein 3, or PCA3 may be incorporated into this tool.

* With the availability of these nomograms, patients considering surgery can be told of the likelihood of finding organ-confined disease, seminal vesicle involvement, or nodal metatases.
    * The Kattan nomogram can calculate the 5-year PFP of surgery and compare it with predictions for other treatment modalities. (The Kattan nomogram can be located online at www.mskcc.org/mskcc/html/10088.cfm.)
    * Desktop and mobile versions are available for downloading. These nomograms also contain functions to determine risk of recurrence after prostatectomy based on pathologic findings.
* **Aside from very advanced age and fixed serious comorbidity, the only contraindications for radical retropubic prostatectomy are compelling evidence of metastatic disease or fixation of the prostate mass to pelvic sidewalls. Once again, a full discussion of the advantages, risks, and complications as well as the likely outcome is extremely important in guiding the patient to the right choice. As always, the guidelines mentioned here are not to be considered absolute. Latitude for patient preferences and surgical judgment must be allowed.**

Laparoscopic Radical Prostatectomy

* Largely supplanted by robotically assisted prostatectomy (see below)

Robotically Assisted Laparoscopic Prostatectomy (RALP)

* A further refinement of the laparoscopic technique
    * Instruments are placed through small port incisions and manipulated by the surgeon at a computer console
    * Advantages
        * Improved visualization due to magnification
        * Instruments provide greater rotational range of motion than human hands
        * Robot dampens adventitious movements by surgeon's hands

- Less bleeding due to increased intra-abdominal pressure on vessels from insufflated air needed for laparoscopic\robotic technique[17]
- Purported to result in less erectile dysfunction and less incontinence, but evidence is lacking
- More rapid recovery because of decreased blood loss and smaller incisions
- Less hospital time—generally one night compared to two nights for open prostatectomy
- Disadvantages
  - Long-term data on complications and cancer control are not yet available.
  - Steep learning curve
  - In a retrospective review of Medicare patients undergoing RALP there was an increased risk of anastomotic strictures and an increased risk of requiring salvage radiotherapy or androgen suppression.[18]

Comment: Most prostatectomies now done in the United States employ robotically assisted techniques. Yet, there are no clinical trials that have proven superiority over standard open prostatectomy for cancer control outcomes or long-term urinary or sexual complications.[19]

Transperineal Radical Prostatectomy[20]

- A rarely used, less invasive approach to prostatectomy for prostate cancer
- Advantages
  - Allows quicker recovery
  - Excellent access to apex allows better visualization of bladder neck
    - Vesicourethral anastomosis is easier
  - Less blood loss
  - Easier to perform in obese patients or in those with prior abdominal surgery
- Disadvantages
  - Lymph node resection not possible
  - Greater risk of impotence because it is more difficult to preserve neurovascular bundles

- Transperineal prostatectomy cannot be performed in patients with severe hip or spine disease that limits or prevents proper positioning.
- *Comment:* Transperineal radical prostatectomy may have a role in limited situations.

Transurethral Resection of the Prostate (TURP)

- TURP is not a curative procedure for prostate cancer.
- Patients found to have prostate cancer in the course of a TURP should be considered for definitive surgery or radiotherapy.
- TURP may be useful as a palliative procedure for a patient whose prostate has not been removed and who has obstructive symptoms.

Postprostatectomy Monitoring

- The serum PSA level should become undetectable within 6 weeks of prostatectomy.
- Persistent or increasing levels after that time correlate with eventual relapse.

Radical Prostatectomy Summary

- Surgical prostatectomy is an effective and safe surgical procedure for selected patients with localized prostate cancer.
- Progression-free survival for favorable risk patients can exceed 90% at 15–20 years depending on risk stratification.
- The increasing use of RALP is not based on data showing superior outcomes or lower complication rates
- The acute perioperative risks are small in healthy patients.
- The risk of erectile dysfunction is significant (40–70%) but highly variable, depending on a number of factors described earlier.
- Most men regain satisfactory urinary control.
- The experience of the surgeon as well as certain tumor characteristics also impact the complication rate.
- These factors may ultimately affect the outcomes more than the type of surgery performed.

■ Radiotherapy Options in the Management of Localized Prostate Cancer

▓ Radiotherapy for prostate currently includes a variety of techniques that have evolved over the past 10–20 years
  • Three-dimensional conformal radiotherapy (3D CRT)
  • Intensity-modulated radiotherapy (IMRT)
  • Image-guided radiotherapy (IGRT)
  • Proton beam therapy
  • Hypofractionated stereotactic radiosurgery (SRS)
  • Low-dose rate permanent seed implants
  • High-dose rate temporary seed implants

▓ Until recently, standard external-beam radiotherapy (EBRT) generally involved bilateral arc rotation or 4-field oblique beams directed at the prostate gland. However, these nonconformal techniques were accompanied by bowel and bladder toxicity that limited the dose delivered to the prostate.

▓ The evolution of newer techniques such as 3D CRT, IMRT, and very recently IMRT with IGRT allows further refinement of the beam and more complex dose distribution, resulting in lower doses to the bladder and bowel despite the delivery of higher doses to the prostate.[21]

EBRT Treatment Details

▓ Imaging is used to define prostate and pelvic anatomy

▓ Treatment plan developed with help of computers

▓ Patients undergoing IGRT require transperineal placement of gold fiducials or electromagnetic transponders so that treatment adjusts for movement of the prostate

▓ Patient is simulated

▓ Treatment is typically given once daily, 5 days per week for approximately 9 weeks, depending on dose.

▓ The radiotherapy is delivered over a few minutes each day.
  • Patients need to allow a total of 1 hour for setup, positioning, examinations, toxicity checks, etc.

▓ Treatment is directed to the entire prostate and the seminal vesicles.

- The inclusion of pelvic lymph nodes is not needed for patients with low-risk disease.
  - Preliminary results of Radiation Therapy Oncology Group (RTOG) 94-13,[22] which compared irradiation of the prostate alone to irradiation of the prostate and pelvic area, suggest a benefit for inclusion of the pelvic nodes in higher-risk disease.
  - Other studies that included patients with low-, intermediate-, and high-risk disease have not demonstrated an advantage for pelvic node irradiation.
- Advantages of EBRT
  - Excellent record of cancer control when adequate doses are delivered (see page 89)
  - Avoids the risks and recovery period associated with surgical prostatectomy
  - Outpatient procedure
  - Less risk of incontinence compared with surgery
  - Less risk of impotence compared with surgery for some patients
- Disadvantages of EBRT
  - Prolonged course of treatment
  - Prostate remains in place
    - Symptoms of BPH may persist or worsen
      - Patients with larger prostate glands (> 40 cc) or very small ones (< 20 cc) may have unacceptable urinary toxicity.
        - Pretreatment androgen-suppressive therapy may be used to reduce prostate size prior to radiotherapy to reduce risk of urinary toxicity.
    - Difficult to monitor for recurrence
      - PSA may fluctuate before reaching nadir.
      - Prostate remains in place and may be difficult to evaluate by DRE because of radiation fibrosis which can cause induration.
      - The use of prostate MRI with endorectal coil may improve ability to monitor after radiotherapy.
    - Salvage surgery more difficult after radiotherapy

- Concerns about radiation-induced secondary tumors in bladder and rectum[23]
  - Isolated cases have been reported, including angiosarcoma and squamous cell carcinoma, but it remains unclear if the overall risk is increased.[24]
  - Radiotherapy may not be feasible for patients with inflammatory bowel disease and those with prior irradiation of the area for other cancers.
- Cancer control with EBRT
  - Comparison with radical prostatectomy is extremely difficult because of
    - Lack of randomized trials—most comparisons are retrospective
    - Downward stage migration in the PSA era
    - Changing radiotherapeutic techniques and dose escalation
    - Mixed patient populations with regards to risk stratification
      - Higher-risk patients tend to be referred for radiotherapy more often than surgery.
    - Variation in the use of salvage therapy at the time of treatment failure
    - Lack of pathologic staging, which allows inadvertant inclusion of patients with higher-risk disease in radiation trials
  - A number of studies showed that cancer control outcomes with radiotherapy were similar to—at least in the short run—those reported for surgery.[25–30]
  - Problems with these trials included:
    - Lack of randomization; most were retrospective
    - A variety of radiotherapy techniques were employed, many of which would be considered outdated in the modern era
    - Doses may have been suboptimal
    - Shorter follow-up times

Table 5-3 Comparative 7-Year Biochemical Relapse-Free Probabilities

7-year Biochemical Relapse-Free Probability	
Radical prostatectomy	76%
External-beam radiation < 72 Gy	47%
External-beam radiation ≥ 72 Gy	82%
Permanent seed implantation	76%
Combination EBRT/PI	77%

- *Comment:* Overall, cancer control outcomes with EBRT are very similar to those seen with radical prostatectomy. Cancer control outcomes are discussed later in reference to IMRT, which had become the de facto standard for EBRT.
- Higher doses of radiotherapy improve relapse-free survival.
  - The development of improved cross-sectional imaging techniques, sophisticated computerized planning, and complex treatment algorithms has allowed dose escalation without a major increase in toxicity to the bowel or bladder.
  - Preliminary data suggest a dose–effect relationship, even for favorable prostate cancers.
    - In 2002 the Memorial Sloan-Kettering Cancer Center (MSKCC) group[31] published their experience with a nonrandomized dose escalation trial. The report was updated in 2008 and included more than 2000 patients. This study included patients with:
      - Clinical stages T1–T3
      - A typical Gleason grade distribution
        - 47% Gleason 6 or less
        - 36% Gleason 7
        - 17% Gleason 8, 9 or 10
      - PSA values of
        - < 10 ng/ml   56%
        - 10–20 ng/ml   26%
        - > 20 NG/ml   18%
      - 52% received neoadjuvant/concurrent androgen-suppressive therapy

- Overall National Comprehensive Cancer Network (NCCN) risk stratification
  - 22% low risk
  - 41% intermediate risk
  - 37% high risk
    - *Comment:* This risk distribution seems higher than what is seen in most surgical series.
- Treatment doses were divided into four groups
  - ≤ 70.2 Gy   17%
  - 75.6 Gy   23%
  - 81.0 Gy   36%
  - 86.4 Gy   24%
- 52% received short-term androgen-suppressive therapy
- Cancer control outcomes: 7-year biochemical recurrence-free survival (bRFS) (actuarial):
  - Low risk: 90%
  - Intermediate risk: 72%
  - High risk: 54%
- Cancer control outcomes: actuarial cause-specific survival
  - Low risk: 99%
  - Intermediate risk: 94%
  - High risk: 81%
    - *Comment:* These outcomes seem similar to those reported after surgery, but length of follow-up is less.

Table 5-4 Actuarial bPFP (5 years)

Dose Level (Gy)	Low-risk bPFP (%)	Intermediate-risk bPFP (%)	High-risk bPFP (%)
64.8–70.2	65	44	22
75.6	86	61	43
81–86.4	96	87	69

- Effect of dose escalation
  - No difference for good-risk patients
  - Intermediate-risk patients had improved bRFS, particularly for those receiving doses of 75.6 Gy compared to 70.2 Gy or less
    - Further escalation beyond 81 Gy did not further improve biochemical outcomes for intermediate-risk patients.
  - High-risk patients had significantly better bRFS if they received 86.4 Gy than those who received 75.6 Gy.
    - Since most of the high-risk patients received androgen-suppressive therapy, it was not possible to attribute the bRFS improvement to the dose of the radiotherapy alone.
  - These results were essentially substantiated by four other randomized trials.[32–35]
- Conclusions
  - Higher radiation doses improve biochemical and metastasis-free survival, at least for intermediate- and high-risk patients.
  - Cancer control outcomes, at least in the short run, seem equivalent to radical prostatectomy.
  - Late GI and GU toxicities reported separately (see below)
- Acute toxicity[14,21]
  - Immediate or short-term toxicity
    - Lower urinary tract symptoms
      - Frequency
      - Nocturia
      - Urgency
      - Dysuria
      - Retention (rare)
    - Rectal symptoms
      - More frequent bowel movements or diarrhea
      - Rectal urgency
      - Exacerbation of hemorrhoids, fissure, etc.
    - Onset as early as week 3 of radiotherapy (or week 3 after seed implants)

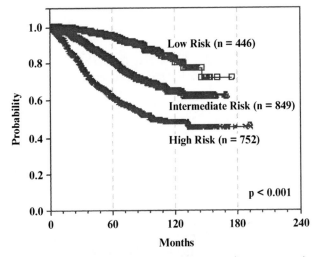

Figure 5-9 PSA relapse free survival outcomes according to prognostic risk group. Reprinted from *Int J Radiation Oncology Bio Phys*, Vol. 71, Issue 4, Zelefsky MJ, et al. Long-term results of conformal radiotherapy for prostate cancer: impact of dose escalation on biochemical tumor control and distant metastases-free survival outcomes, pages 1028–33, copyright 2008, with permission from Elsevier.

- May last several months or up to 1 year
- Usually managed symptomatically
  - Loperamide or diphenoxylate plus atropine for diarrhea
  - Sitz baths and hydrocortisone ointment for hemorrhoids
  - Phenazopyridine or alpha-blockers for urinary symptoms
  - Anti-inflammatory agents
- Fatigue, generally mild to moderate, is common toward the end of the treatment course.
- Late toxicity (3 months or longer after completion of EBRT)
  - Urinary symptoms
    - Dysuria, frequency, urgency
    - Hematuria due to radiation cystitis
    - Urethral stricture
      - Surgical intervention rarely required
  - Rectal symptoms
    - Diarrhea
    - Urgency
    - Bleeding due to proctitis

- Rectal discharge
- Anal stricture
- Sexual dysfunction
  - Potency is initially preserved in approximately three quarters of men, but erectile function declines with time.
  - At 5 years, the risk of erectile dysfunction rate is 33–61%[36]
  - Dry ejaculate
  - Infertility
    - Men anticipating radiotherapy for localized prostate cancer should consider sperm banking if they want more children.
  - Secondary cancers
  - The MSKCC group reported on late rectal and urinary toxicities after 3D CRT and IMRT.[37]
    - Patient characteristics
      - 1571 patients with T1–T3 treated with either 3D CRT or IMRT to between 66 and 81 Gy
        - All IMRT was given to 81 Gy
      - 43% received androgen-suppressive therapy
      - Median follow-up 8 years
    - Acute (short-term) toxicity
      - Grade 2 or higher rectal toxicity
        - IMRT 3%
        - 3D CRT 1%
      - Grade 2 or higher urinary toxicity 16%
        - Higher in those receiving IMRT at 81 Gy
    - Late GI toxicity (rectal bleeding or discharge)
      - Onset between 4 and 102 months
      - Grade 2 or higher 6%
        - 91% resolved within 2 years
      - Grade 3: 1%
      - Only one patient developed grade 4 toxicity, and this was in the setting of pre-existing inflammatory bowel disease.
      - Actuarial risk of grade 2 or higher rectal toxicity at 10 years was 9%.
      - Less late GI toxicity with IMRT (5%) than with 3D CRT (13%)

- Late GU toxicity
  - Median time to onset: 30 months
  - Grade 2: 8%
    - Mainly frequency and urgency
    - Incontinence rare
    - 81% resolved with median time of 7 months
  - Grade 3: 3%
    - Mainly urethral strictures requiring TURP
  - Dose important
  - 20% late GU toxicity for those receiving 81 Gy (IMRT) compared to 12% with lower doses.

Table 5-5 Late Rectal and Urinary Toxicity after IMRT

Grade	Rectal Toxicity (%)	Urinary Toxicity (%)
0	85.2	62.0
1	12.6	25.9
2	1.4	11.5
3	0.8	0.6
4	0.0	0.0

- Sexual outcomes were reported in a separate publication analyzing patients who received 81 Gy of IMRT[38]
  - 49% of men who were sexually active before treatment developed erectile dysfunction
    - IMRT alone: 43%
    - IMRT plus short course of androgen-suppressive therapy: 57%
- No secondary cancers were observed in this cohort, but follow-up time is relatively short.
  - *Comment:* The MSKCC group is now routinely using IMRT/IGRT with doses to 86.4 Gy in 48 fractions for all patients, including those with favorable risk factors.

Image-Guided Radiotherapy

- A form of IMRT in which imaging is used to reduce errors related to prostate movement in between and during radiotherapy sessions
- Transrectally inserted gold fiducials allow precise tracking of prostate position by CT.
- The Calypso system uses implanted electromagnetic transponders to continuously monitor and correct for prostate movement during the actual delivery of the radiotherapy.
- No long-term results have been reported regarding either effectiveness of treatment or reduction of side effects.

Proton Therapy

- A form of external radiotherapy using protons instead of photons
- Interaction with tissue is different
  - Lower dose as proton enters body
  - Easier to set the tissue depth that receives the maximal dose (Bragg's peak)
  - No exit dose beyond peak[39]
- Requires cyclotron
  - Much more expensive than IMRT
- No proven benefit over photons for prostate cancer.

Posttreatment Follow-Up

- Nadir PSA level is an independent variable for long-term biochemical freedom from progression.
- It may take 1–2 years for nadir to be reached, and PSA may fluctuate before reaching nadir.
  - PSA nadir level of 1 ng/ml or greater: 5-year PFP of 30%
  - PSA nadir level of less than 1 ng/ml: 5-year PFP of 83%[40]
- Failure is defined by the American Society of Therapeutic Radiology as 2.0 ng/mL above nadir[41]
- Clinicians should be aware that PSA levels may "bounce" or increase within the first 2–3 years after treatment. The cause is unknown.

Interstitial Prostate Brachytherapy (Seed Implants)

- The idea that higher doses of radiation, and consequently improved outcomes, could be achieved by the permanent implantation of radioactive seeds is not a new one.
- Early results were disappointing because of the inaccuracy of free-hand open retropubic insertion techniques.
- The development of transperineal ultrasound and more recently computer-guided permanent percutaneous seed implantation has allowed higher doses of radiation to be delivered (115–145 Gy), resulting in favorable cancer control outcomes with acceptable toxicity for selected patients.
- It should be noted that a given dose delivered by EBRT is not equivalent radiobiologically to the same dose administered by brachytherapy. Brachytherapy as a single modality or a combination of brachytherapy and EBRT is becoming more and more popular for the treatment of localized prostate cancer.
- Advantages
  - Prostate motion not an issue since dose implanted directly into prostate
  - Doses higher than those given with IMRT
  - Less dose to surrounding normal tissues
  - Complete treatment delivered in one outpatient session (low-dose rate) or during short inpatient stay (high-dose rate)
- Disadvantages
  - Requires anesthesia
  - Not suitable for all patients (see below)
    - High-risk patients
      - Periprostatic tissue, seminal vesicles, and lymph nodes may not be adequately treated with implant alone.
      - High-risk patients should be considered for either EBRT alone, EBRT in combination with LDR seed implants, or HDR seed implants.
    - Patients with very large (> 100 cc) or very small (< 10 cc) prostates
    - Patients with anatomical variations in pubic arch rendering implantation of entire gland difficult or impossible.

- Occasional seed migration with unknown clinical significance (LDR seed implant only)
- Close contact with children under 18 and pregnant women must be avoided for 1–2 months, depending on isotope used (LDR seed implant only)
- Bowel and bladder toxicity
- Acute urinary symptoms more pronounced than with EBRT

Low-Dose Rate Transperineal Permanent Seed Implants (TPSI)

- Technique
  - Outpatient transperineal insertion of radioactive seeds containing either ^{125}I or [103]Pd (**Figure 5-10**)
    - Permanent transperineal implant techniques continue to evolve beyond free-hand insertion. Most implants are performed using ultrasound guidance.
      - The MSKCC group is currently using real-time planning techniques, which involve intraoperative computer-optimized ultrasound-guided placement of radioactive seeds, rather than preplanning techniques.[42]

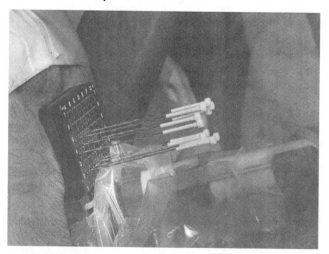

Figure 5-10 Transperineal ultrasound-guided seed implantation. Reprinted from *Int J Radiation Oncology Bio Phys*, Vol. 53, Issue 5, Zelefsky MJ, et al. High-dose IMRT for PCa, pages 1111–6, copyright 2002, with permission from Elsevier.

- Intraoperative computer-optimized planning results in improved dose distribution, less urinary toxicity, and improved bPFP compared with preplanning techniques.[43]
- Type of radioactive implant
  - ^{125}I
    - Higher dose (~144 Gy)
    - Slower dose rate (~7 cGy/h)
    - Half-life of 60 days
    - More commonly used in slower-growing, lower-grade tumors for monotherapy
  - ^{103}Pd
    - Lower dose (115–125 Gy)
    - More rapid dose rate (18–20 cGy/h)
    - Half-life of 17 days
    - Favored by some for more aggressive, higher-grade tumors
  - In a study of patients treated with ^{125}I versus those treated with ^{103}Pd, Peschel[44] noted very similar 5-year bPFP rates for all patients. Less urinary toxicity was observed in the Palladium group.

Table 5-6 5-year bPFP

Risk level	^{125}I (%)	^{103}Pd (%)
Low	92	92
Intermediate and high	72	74

- Case selection[45,46]
  - Disagreement still exists among experienced groups as to criteria for either selecting or excluding brachytherapy as primary therapy. The following are general guidelines:
    - Good candidates[47]
      - Clinical stage T1c–T2b
      - Gleason score of 6 or low volume Gleason 7 cancers
      - PSA level of less than 10 ng/ml
      - Low risk determined by nomogram

- Prostate gland size ≥ 20 cc and < 50 cc
  - Patients with glands measuring 50–100 cc may have a response to cytoreductive hormone therapy sufficient to allow brachytherapy.
  - Patients with gland sizes greater than 100 cc are unlikely to have enough shrinkage to allow this approach.
  - Very large prostate glands may extend beneath the pubic arch, limiting the ability to implant the entire gland.
- Relative contraindications
  - Patients with clinical stage > T2b, extensive Gleason 7, or high grade (Gleason 8–10), neuroendocrine or small cell cancers
  - Orthopedic problems that limit hip flexion
  - Prior TURP
    - May increase risk of urinary toxicity
  - Tumor involvement of the transitional zone
  - Median lobe hypertrophy
  - Severe preexisting irritative or obstructive symptoms
    - International Prostate Symptom Score (IPSS) of greater than 15
  - Inflammatory bowel disease
  - These relative contraindications, when present, may result in increased toxicity or suboptimal outcome.
- Absolute contraindications
  - Severe fixed comorbidity that either precludes anesthesia or significantly limits life expectancy
  - Very high-risk disease
    - Gleason score of 8–10, neuroendocrine or small cell cancers
    - T stage higher than T2b
    - PSA level of 10 ng/ml or greater

- Cancer control outcomes
  - A number of centers have published favorable results that are comparable, at least in the short run, to radical prostatectomy. These results are summarized in a number of reports.[46–49]
  - In general, bPFP rates at 5 years are favorable
    - Low-risk disease: 85–96%[50]
      - 93% bRFS at 8 years
    - Intermediate-risk disease: 67–82%
    - High-risk disease: 52–65%
  - In a non-randomized study involving favorable risk patients, the Memorial Sloan-Kettering Cancer Center group compared cancer control outcomes and toxicity in 448 consecutive patients receiving brachytherapy (144 Gy)with 281 patients receiving intensity-modulated radiotherapy (81 Gy).[51]
  - At 7 years biochemical relapse-free survival was similar in both groups
  - Brachytherapy 95% vs IMRT 89% p = 0.004
  - Late grade 2 gastrointestinal (rectal) toxicity was slightly worse for the brachytherapy group 5.1% vs 1.4% in the IMRT group p = 0.02
  - Late Grade 2 urinary toxicity was slightly higher for the brachytherapy group 15.6% vs 4.3% p < 0.0001
  - Late Grade 3 urinary and rectal toxicity was very rare (< 2.2%) and similar in both groups.

Note: **The lack of truly long-term data, even for favorable risk patients, has been used as an argument against brachytherapy, particularly for younger men who have a longer period of time at risk. Proponents of brachytherapy argue that the data are maturing, with 10-year and even 15-year data becoming available. They point out that late relapse is rare and that comparison with surgery or EBRT is treacherous given the rapid changes in treatment techniques and the downward stage migration in the PSA era.**

- Complications
  - Short-term (< 6 months) toxicities
    - Irritative urinary symptoms: frequency, dysuria, and urgency
    - Urinary retention (10%)
      - Typically self-limited
      - Managed by self-catheterization in most cases
    - Diarrhea
    - Rectal frequency/urgency or rectal spasms
    - Exacerbation of hemorrhoids, fissures, etc.
  - Long-term toxicities
    - Serious toxicity (grade 4–5) is unusual
    - 2–18% develop late, grade 2–3 toxicity[48]
      - Urinary
        - Incontinence (1–6.6%; more common in elderly patients)[52]
        - Urethral stricture
        - Cystitis/urethritis and urinary bleeding
      - Rectal
        - Proctitis (5%)
          - Usually characterized by minor bleeding
          - Rarely requires surgical intervention or transfusion
      - Sexual dysfunction
        - Impotence (14–38% in men with no preexisting erectile dysfunction)[49]
- Follow-up after brachytherapy
  - Because the definition of failure varies, the interpretation of results is difficult.
    - Nadir plus 2.0 ng/mL
    - Absolute PSA value greater than or equal to 2 with three increases in PSA of 0.5 ng/mL each
  - PSA bounce
    - The serum PSA level may increase slightly over a 12–30-month period.
    - This occurs in approximately one-third of patients without signifying relapse.[46]

EBRT Plus Seed Implant

- Disappointing results with brachytherapy alone for higher-risk disease has led to the use of combined brachytherapy and EBRT.
- Advantages
  - Offers another option to patients with higher-risk disease
  - Delivers higher doses of radiation to the prostate
  - Disease extending beyond the prostate capsule to include the seminal vesicles and pelvic lymph nodes may be controlled by the EBRT.
  - Shorter course of therapy compared with EBRT alone
- Disadvantages
  - Longer course of therapy compared with brachytherapy alone
  - Some patients are not candidates for brachytherapy.
  - Potential for increased toxicity
- Cancer control outcomes
  - The absence of randomized controlled trials and the short follow-up in most series limit the evaluation of efficacy.
  - Febles et al.[53] reviewed several reports indicating excellent cancer control with combined EBRT and brachytherapy in patients with intermediate- or high-risk disease. Actuarial bPFP rates of almost 80% were seen for 3–10 years. Urinary and bowel toxicity were similar to what has been described for single modality therapy. Potency was preserved in approximately 75% of patients.
  - Longer-term data was recently presented by Sylvester et al.[54] from Seattle. In this report, 223 patients received either ^{125}I or [103]Pd with neoadjuvant EBRT. Of these patients, 27% had low-risk, 41% had intermediate-risk, and 32% had high-risk disease.

Table 5-7 Cancer Control Outcomes for Combined EBRT and Permanent Seed Implants

Risk Level	15-year bRFS (%)	Disease-specific Survival (%)
Low	86	93
Intermediate	72	86
High	47	59

- These data suggest that outcomes for low- and intermediate-risk disease are similar to those achieved with prostatectomy, EBRT, or brachytherapy alone. Improved therapy is needed for patients with high-risk disease who seem to do poorly in general. This issue is addressed in the following chapter.

High-Dose Rate Temporary Seed Implants

- The use of HDR iridium (Ir 192), either alone or in conjunction with EBRT, is receiving renewed attention, particularly in high-risk disease.
  - A radioactive source is inserted through an attached cable into each of several implanted catheters and allowed to "dwell" for a predetermined period of time.
  - The first fraction of HDR is given the first day.
  - The catheters are left in place, and one or two fractions are delivered.
  - At the completion of therapy, the catheters are removed and the patient is discharged, without radioactive material in his prostate.
  - May be used alone or in conjunction with EBRT
  - Advantages[39]
    - No radiation safety issues posttreatment as seeds are removed
    - Better coverage of extraprostatic disease without risk of seed migration
  - Disadvantages
    - Short hospital stay may be required
    - No long-term data on efficacy or toxicity since this is a relatively recent development
    - Requires anesthesia and immobilization during implant insertion

- Cancer control outcomes
  - 8 year bRFS
    - Intermediate risk: 87%
    - High risk: 69%[55]
- The role for this modality remains to be defined.

Note: It should be understood that intermediate- and high-risk patients typically will also undergo androgen-suppressive therapy (see Chapter 6).

Hypofractionated External-Beam Radiotherapy

- Stereotactic radiosurgery (Gamma Knife, CyberKnife)
  - Treatment given in 4–5 fractions, higher dose per fraction
  - Short-term outcome and toxicity data are similar to other radiotherapy techniques but long-term data not yet available.[56,57]

Other Nonsurgical Approaches to Localized Prostate Cancer That Are Unproven

- Cryotherapy
- Microwave ablation
- High-frequency ultrasound
- Focal therapy with radiation or cryosurgery
  - Requires "saturation" biopsy to rule out more diffuse involvement of the prostate
  - Clinical trials underway for patients with small volume, low Gleason score disease on initial biopsy
- The value of and exact indications for these procedures remain undefined.

■ Noncurative Approaches to Localized Prostate Cancer

Androgen-Suppressive Therapy (AST)

- The use of androgen-suppressive therapy alone in patients with localized asymptomatic prostate cancer—as a compromise option for men who decline surgery or radiotherapy or men who are not candidates for definitive therapy because of advanced age or comorbidities—should be discouraged as survival may be less than for those undergoing watchful waiting.

- On the other hand, androgen-suppressive therapy alone may be reasonable in this setting if the prostate tumor is very large or causing urinary or rectal obstructive symptoms or pain.

Watchful Waiting

- Watchful waiting is a conservative strategy for asymptomatic men whose life expectancy is expected to be very short because of very advance age or serious comorbidities.
- In this strategy patients are followed without aggressive diagnostic or therapeutic intervention until and unless they become symptomatic at which time palliative rather than curative therapy is instituted.
- Most men in this situation will die of other illnesses before treatment of their prostate cancer becomes necessary.

Active Surveillance

- Because many of the early prostate cancers diagnosed by PSA level (and even by DRE) have very little short-term potential to spread or pose a threat to patients harboring them, and because treatment is commonly associated with a decrease in quality of life, active surveillance is an attractive option for some men. Unfortunately, reliable methods to distinguish indolent cancers from those needing treatment do not yet exist.
- Advantages
  * Avoids acute risks and long-term toxicities of treatment
  * Preserves quality of life
  * Many men will never become symptomatic and will go on to die of other causes.
- Disadvantages
  * More anxiety provoking for many (but not all) men
  * Possibility of needle biopsy underestimating extent of tumor
  * Possibility of more aggressive cancer being present than is identified on needle biopsy
  * Continued possibility that cancer will advance locally or spread, resulting in symptomatic prostate cancer or death from the disease

- Attempts at curative therapy at time of progression may be associated with worse outcome and more side effects.
- Requires frequent medical visits, blood tests, and repeat biopsies (see below)
- The goal of active surveillance remains curative but seeks to individualize management, deferring definitive therapy until there are changes that suggest a higher risk of progression.
  - This strategy involves close follow-up, with PSA level determinations every 3–4 months for the first 2 years and every 6 months thereafter.
  - Biopsies are repeated in the first 6–12 months and again at 12–18-month intervals.
  - Potentially curative treatment may be offered if
    - The PSA rapidly increases.
    - DRE or imaging reveals local progression of disease.
    - Rebiopsy reveals increase in Gleason score or more extensive involvement of the biopsy cores.
    - The patient becomes symptomatic.
  - Patients chosen for this strategy should be eligible for definitive therapy and have low to intermediate risk factors.
    - NCCN guidelines suggest that active surveillance is an option for men with
      - Very good-risk disease and a life expectancy of less than 20 years
        - Clinical stage T1c
        - Gleason score 6 or less
        - PSA equal to or less than 10 ng/mL
        - No more than three positive biopsy cores
          - No core more than 50% involved
        - PSA density < 0.15 ng/mL/g
      - Low-risk disease and a life expectancy of less than 10 years
        - T1–T2a
        - Gleason score less than or equal to 6
        - PSA less than 10

- The feasibility of active surveillance was shown by Choo et al.[58] in 2002. In a nonrandomized trial, 206 patients with localized prostate cancer were followed prospectively.
  * Criteria for participation included
    - Clinical stage lower than T3
    - Gleason score of 7 or less
    - PSA levels of 15 ng/ml or less
  * Median age was 70 years (range: 49–84 years)
    - Definitive treatment was offered if any of the following occurred
    - PSA doubling time was less than 24 months
    - Repeat biopsy upgraded the Gleason score
    - Patient developed clinical symptoms
  * At a median follow-up of 29 months
    - 137 men (66%) remained on observation.
    - 35 men (17%) progressed by the study criteria.
    - The remainder were removed from the study for a variety of reasons, including patient request, protocol violation, and death from other causes.
    - Actuarial probability of remaining on protocol at 4 years was 48%.
    - Actuarial probability of remaining progression free at 4 years was 67%.
  * Although this study demonstrated the feasibility of active surveillance, there were no long-term data for progression-free probability, disease-specific survival, or overall survival. The group from Johns Hopkins recently updated their experience with active surveillance.[59]
    - 769 men with very low-risk prostate cancer
      * Clinical stage T1c
      * PSA density < 0.15 ng/ml
      * No more than two positive biopsy cores
      * No more than 50% involvement of any core
    - Median follow-up 2.7 years (range 0.01–15 years)

- Median intervention-free survival was 6.5 years
  - 81% free of intervention at 2 years
  - 59% free of intervention at 5 years
  - 41% free of intervention at 10 years
- One-third of the patients underwent curative intervention at a median of 2.2 years, most for changes on repeat biopsy
- 9.4% of the men undergoing definitive treatment had PSA relapse within 2 years of treatment
- None of the patients developed metastatic disease or died of prostate cancer.
- Problems with this study are relatively short follow-up time and use of PSA posttreatment as a surrogate for long-term survival
  - A number of other non randomized trials and two randomized trials are currently underway, but long-term results are not yet available.
  - Common to these trials are the exclusion of higher risk patients by virtue of PSA, Gleason scores, number of positive cores, percentage of involvement of the cores, and in some cases PSA kinetics or density.
  - Time to intervention is roughly similar, and with very short term follow up, biochemical freedom from progression rates seem similar to those who undergo therapy without having treatment deferred.[60]
    - Comment on Active Surveillance
      - Active surveillance should be considered for selected patients with favorable risk prostate cancer with the caveat that the long term impact of the delay in definitive therapy is not known. That could be a relatively minor consideration in older men, but it becomes important in younger men, who are most concerned about side effects of therapy.

■ Summary: Management of Localized Prostate Cancer

■ The prognosis for most men diagnosed with localized prostate cancer is excellent.

■ It must be emphasized that there is no strong evidence for superiority of any treatment modality over any other.

■ In choosing treatment for early prostate cancer, individual preferences and values must be considered.

  • Some men will choose maximum confidence in terms of outcome, accepting whatever toxicity develops.

  • Others prefer to avoid specific toxicities and choose treatment that may have less of a chance of curing the cancer.

  • A surprising number of patients include salvage therapy possibilities in their decision-making process. This should be discouraged for reasons to be discussed in the Biochemical Failure and Salvage Therapy chapter (Chapter 7, pp. 137).

  • The following are recommendations for management of localized disease. They are only guidelines and should not supersede the clinical judgment of the treating physicians or the informed choice of the patient. The management of intermediate- and high-risk prostate cancer is discussed in Chapter 6.

  • Radical prostatectomy should be considered in men with localized prostate cancer who are physiologically fit.

    ■ Other options should be considered in men over 70 unless they are in extraordinarily good health.

  • Even high-risk patients may benefit from prostatectomy.

  • Robotically assisted surgery is becoming more common, but there are no data to support the notion that outcomes are better.

  • Radiotherapy is a reasonable option for treatment of localized prostate cancer.

  • The current standard for external-beam therapy (EBRT) involves intensity/modulated techniques with image guidance (IMRT\IGRT).

  • Dose escalation to as much as 86.4 Gy has been shown to improve survival without a major change in long-term bowel or bladder toxicity.

- Low-dose rate transperineal permanent seed implantation with either Iodine 125 or Palladium 103 is another option for favorable-risk prostate cancer.
- The combination of EBRT plus seed implantation is becoming more common, although the exact indications remain unclear.
- High-dose rate temporary seed implants may have a role particularly in patients with higher-risk disease.
- Androgen-suppressive therapy alone as treatment for localized prostate cancer should be discouraged unless the patient is symptomatic and is not a candidate for surgery or any form of radiation therapy.
- Watchful waiting is appropriate in asymptomatic men with very limited life expectancy.
- Active surveillance is a reasonable option for men with low-risk disease and a life expectancy of less than 20 years.
- The long-term safety of active surveillance has not been established.
- In recent years many new techniques have been marketed without long-term safety or efficacy data. They should be considered experimental.

The author would like to recognize the advice and suggestions of Drs. Michael J. Zelefsky and Marissa Kollmeier that contributed to the radiotherapy section of this chapter.

■ References

1. Catalona WJ, Ramos CG, Carvalhal GF. Contemporary results of anatomic radical prostatectomy. *CA Cancer J Clin.* 1999;49:282–296.
2. Hull GW, Rabbani F, Abbas F, Wheeler TM, Kattan MW, Scardino PT. Cancer control with radical prostatectomy alone in 1,000 consecutive patients. *J Urol.* 2002;167(pt 1):528–534.
3. Pound CR, Partin AW, Epstein JI, Walsh PC. Prostate-specific antigen after anatomic radical retropubic prostatectomy. Patterns of recurrence and cancer control. *Urol Clin North Am.* 1997;24:395–406.

4. Catalona WJ, Partin AW, Slawin KM, et al. Use of the percentage of free prostate-specific antigen to enhance differentiation of prostate cancer from benign prostatic disease: a prospective multicenter clinical trial. *JAMA.* 1998;279: 1542–1547.

5. Zincke H, Oesterling JE, Blute ML, Bergstralh EJ, Myers RP, Barrett DM. Long-term (15 years) results after radical prostatectomy for clinically localized (stage T2c or lower) prostate cancer. *J Urol.* 1994;152:1850–1857.

6. Bianco F, et al. Fifteen year cancer-specific and PSA progression free probabilities after radical abstract prostatectomy. In 99th American Urological Association Annual Meeting. *J Urol.* 2004;171(Suppl 4).

7. Ohori M, Kattan M, Scardino PT, Wheeler TM. Radical prostatectomy for carcinoma of the prostate. *Mod Pathol.* 2004;17:349–359.

8. Stephenson AJ, Kattan MW, Eastham JA, et al. Prostate cancer-specific mortality after radical prostatectomy for patients treated in the prostate-specific antigen era. *J Clin Onc.* 2009;27:4300–5.

9. Potter SR, Partin AW. Surgical therapy of clinically localized prostate cancer: rationale, patient selection, and outcomes. In: Kantoff PW, Carroll PR, D'Amico AV, eds. *Prostate Cancer: Principles and Practice.* Philadelphia: Lippincott Williams and Wilkins; 2002:307–316.

10. Carlsson S, Adolfsson J, Bratt O, et al Nationwide population based study on 30 day mortality after readial prostatectomy in Sweden. *Scan J Urol Nephrol.* 2009;43(5) 350–6.

11. Lepor H, Nieder AM, Ferrandino MN. Intraoperative and postoperative complications of radical retropubic prostatectomy in a consecutive series of 1,000 cases. *J Urol.* 2001; 166:1729–1733.

12. Eastham JA, Scardino PT. Radical prostatectomy. In: Campbell MF, Retik AB, Vaughn ED, Walsh PC, eds. *Campbell's Urology.* 7th ed. Philadelphia: WB Saunders; 1998:2547–2564.

13. Walsh PC. Anatomic radical retropubic prostatectomy. In: Campbell MF, Retik AB, Vaughn ED, Walsh PC, eds. *Campbell's Urology.* Philadelphia: WB Saunders; 1998:2565–2588.

14. Scher H, Leibel SA, Fuks Z, Cordon-Cardo C, Scardino PT. Cancer of the prostate. In: DeVita VT, Hellman S, Rosenberg SA, eds. *Cancer: Principles and Practice of Oncology.* 7th ed. Philadelphia: Lippincott Williams and Wilkins; 2005:1192–1259.

15. Catalona WJ, Carvalhal GE, Mager DE, Smith DS. Potency, continence and complication rates in 1,870 consecutive radical retropubic prostatectomies. *J Urol*. 1999;162:433–438.

16. Potosky AL, Davis WW, Hoffman RM, et al. Five year outcomes after prostatectomy or radiotherapy for prostate cancer: the Prostate Cancer Outcomes Study. *J Natl Cancer Inst*. 2004;96:1358–1367.

17. Menon M, Tewari A, Peabody JO, et al. Vattikuti Institute prostatectomy, a technique of robotic radical prostatectomy for management of localized carcinoma of the prostate: experience of over 1100 cases. *Urol Clin North Am*. 2004;31:701–717.

18. Hu JC, Wang Q, Pashos CL, et al. Utilization of outcomes of minimally invasive radical prostatectomy. *J Clin Oncol*. 2008 May 10;26(14):2278–84.

19. Kang, DC et al. Low quality of evidence for robot-assisted laparoscopic prostatectomy: results of a systematic review of the published literature. *Eur Urol* (2010), doi: 10.1016/j.eururo.2010.01.034

20. Linton KD, Hamdy FC. Early diagnosis and surgical management of prostate cancer. *Cancer Treat Rev*. 2003;29:151–160.

21. Michalski JM. External beam radiation therapy: conventional and conformal. In: Kantoff PW, Carroll PR, D'Amico AV, eds. *Prostate Cancer: Principles and Practice*. Philadelphia: Lippincott Williams and Wilkins; 2002;317–335.

22. Roberts T, Roach M III. The evolving role of pelvic radiation therapy. *Semin Radiat Oncol*. 2003;13:109–120.

23. Baxter NN, Tepper JE, Durham SB, Rothenberger DA, Virnig BA. Increased risk of rectal cancer after prostate radiation: a population-based study. *Gastroenterology*. 2005;128:819–824.

24. Pickles T, Phillips N. The risk of second malignancy in men with prostate cancer treated with or without radiation in British Columbia, 1984–2000. *Radiother Oncol*. 2002;65:145–151.

25. Kupelian PA, Potters L, Khuntia D, et al. Radical prostatectomy, external beam radiotherapy < 72 Gy, external beam radiotherapy > or = 72 Gy, permanent seed implantation, or combined seeds/external beam radiotherapy for stage T1–T2 prostate cancer. *Int J Radiat Oncol Biol Phys*. 2004;58:25–33.

26. Shipley WU, Thames HD, Sandler HM, et al. Radiation therapy for clinically localized prostate cancer: a multi-institutional pooled analysis. *JAMA*. 1999;281:1598–1604.

27. D'Amico AV, Whittington R, Malkowicz SB, et al. Biochemical outcome after radical prostatectomy or external beam radiation therapy for patients with clinically localized prostate carcinoma in the prostate specific antigen era. *Cancer.* 2002;95:281–286.

28. Vicini FA, Martinez A, Hanks G, et al. An interinstitutional and interspecialty comparison of treatment outcome data for patients with prostate carcinoma based on predefined prognostic categories and minimum follow-up. *Cancer.* 2002;95:2126–2135.

29. Roach M III, Lu J, Pilepich MV, et al. Long-term survival after radiotherapy alone: Radiation Therapy Oncology Group prostate cancer trials. *J Urol.* 1999;161:864–868.

30. Nilsson S, Norlen BJ, Widmark A. A systematic overview of radiation therapy effects in prostate cancer. *Acta Oncol.* 2004;43:316–381.

31. Zelefsky MJ, Fuks Z, Hunt M, et al. High-dose intensity modulated radiation therapy for prostate cancer: early toxicity and biochemical outcome in 772 patients. *Int J Radiat Oncol Biol Phys.* 2002;53:1111–1116.

32. Pollack A, Zagars GK, Smith LG. Preliminary results of a randomized radiotherapy dose escalation study comparing 70 Gy with 78 Gy for prostate cancer. *J Clin Oncol.* 2000;18:3904–3911.

33. Zietman AL, DeSilvio ML, Slater JD, et al. Comparison of conventional dose vs. high dose conformal radiation therapy in clinically localized adenocarcinoma of the prostate: a randomized trial. *JAMA.* 2005;294:1233–1239.

34. Peeters STH, Heemsbergen WD, Kper PCM, et al. Dose response in radiotherapy for localized prostate cancer: results of the Dutch multicenter randomized Phase III trial comparing 68 Gy of radiotherapy with 78 Gy. *J Clin Oncol.* 2006; 24: 1990–1996.

35. Dearnaley DP, Sydes MR, Graham JD, et al. Escalated dose versus standard dose conformal radiotherapy in prostate cancer: First results from the MRC RT 01 randomised controlled trial. *Lancet Oncol.* 2007;9:474–487.

36. Shipley WU, Zietman A, Hanks GE, et al. Treatment related sequelae following external beam radiation for prostate cancer: a review with an update in patients with stages T1 and T2 tumor. *J Urol.* 1994;152(pt 2):1799–1805.

37. Zelefsky MJ, Levin EJ, Hunt M, et al. Incidence of late rectal and urinary toxicities after three dimensional conformal radiotherapy and intensity modulated radiotherapy for localized prostate cancer. *Int J Radiat Oncol Biol Phys.* 2008; 70(4):1124–1129.

38. Zelefsky M, Chan H, Hunt M, et al. Long term outcome of high dose intensity modulated radiation therapy for patients with localized prostate cancer. *J Urol.* 2006;176:1415–1419.

39. Biagioli MC, Hoffe SE. Emerging technologies in prostate cancer radiation therapy: improving the therapeutic window. *Cancer Control.* 2010;17(4):223–232.

40. Kavadi VS, Zagars GK, Pollack A. Serum prostate-specific antigen after radiation therapy for clinically localized prostate cancer: prognostic implications. *Int J Radiat Oncol Biol Phys.* 1997;30:279–287.

41. American Society for Therapeutic Radiology and Oncology Consensus Panel. Consensus statement: guidelines for PSA following radiation therapy. *Int J Radiat Oncol Biol Phys.* 1997;37:1035–1041.

42. Nag S, Ciezki JP, Cormack R, et al. Intraoperative planning and evaluation of permanent prostate brachytherapy: report of American Brachytherapy Society. *Int J Radiat Oncol Biol Phys.* 2001;51:1422–1430.

43. Zelefsky MJ, Yamada Y, Marion C, et al. Improved conformality and decreased toxicity with intraoperative computer-optimized transperineal ultrasound-guided prostate brachytherapy. *Int J Radiat Oncol Biol Phys.* 2003;55:956–963.

44. Peschel RE, Colberg JW, Chen Z, Nath R, Wilson LD. Iodine 125 versus palladium 103 implants for prostate cancer: clinical outcomes and complications. *Cancer J.* 2004;10:170–174.

45. Merrick GS, Wallner KE, Butler WM. Patient selection for prostate brachytherapy: more myth than fact. *Oncology.* 2004;18:445–452.

46. Langley SE, Laing RW. Iodine seed prostate brachytherapy: an alternative first-line choice for early prostate cancer. *Prostate Cancer Prostatic Dis.* 2004;7:201–207.

47. Nag S, Beyer D, Friedland J, et al. American brachytherapy society recommendations for transperineal permanent brachytherapy of prostate cancer. *Int J Radiat Oncol Biol Phys.* 1999; 44(4): 789–799.

48. Peschel RE, Colberg JW. Surgery, brachytherapy, and external-beam radiotherapy for early prostate cancer. *Lancet Oncol.* 2003;4:233–241.

49. Quaranta BP, Marks LB, Anscher MS. Comparing radical prostatectomy and brachytherapy for localized prostate cancer. *Oncology.* 2004;18:1289–1302.

50. Zelefsky MJ, Kuban DA, Levy LB, et al. Multi-institutional analysis of long term outcome for stages T1–T2 prostate cancer treated with permanent seed implantation. *Int J Radiat Oncol Biol Phys.* 2007:67(2): 327–333.

51. Zelefsky MJ, Yamada Y, and Pei X, et al. Comparison of tumor control and toxicity outcomes of high dose intensity-modulated radiotherapy and brachytherapy for favorable risk prostate cancer. *Urology.* 2011;77(4): 986–90.

52. Benoit RM, Naslund MJ, Cohen JK. Complications after prostate brachytherapy in the Medicare population. *Urology.* 2000;55:91–96.

53. Febles C, Valicenti RK. Combining external beam radiotherapy with prostate brachytherapy: issues and rationale. *Urology.* 2004;64:855–861.

54. Sylvester JE, Blasko JC, Grimm PD, Meier R, Spiegel JF, Malmgren JA, et al. Fifteen year follow up of the first cohort of localized prostate cancer patients treated with brachytherapy. *Proc Am Soc Clin Oncol.* 2004;23:397a. Abstract 4567.

55. Demanes DJ, Rodriguez RR, Schour L, et al. High dose rate intensity modulated brachytherapy for prostate cancer: California endocurietherapy's 10 year results. *Int J Radioat Oncol Biol Phys.* 2005;61(5):1306–1316.

56. Madsen BL, HIS RA, Pham HT, et al. Stereotactic hypo-fractionated accurate radiotherapy of the prostate (SHARP), 33.5 Gy in five fractions for localized disease: first clinical trial results. *Int J Radiat Biol Phys.* 2007; 67(4): 1099–1105.

57. King CR, Brooks JD, Gill H, et al. Stereotactic body radiotherapy for localized prostate cancer: interim results of prospective phase II clinical trial. *Int J Radiat Oncolo Biol Phys.* 2009;73(4):1043–1048.

58. Choo R, Klotz L, Danjoux C, et al. Feasibility study: watchful waiting for localized low to intermediate grade prostate carcinoma with selective delayed intervention based on prostate specific antigen, histological and/or clinical progression. *J Urol.* 2002;167:1664–1669.

59. Tosoian JJ, Trock BJ, Landis P, et al. Active surveillance program for prostate cancer: an update of the Johns Hopkins experience. *J Clin Onc.* 2011;(29) 16: 2185–90.

60. Cooperberg MR, Carroll PR and Klotz L. Active Surveillance for Prostate Cancer: Progress and Promise. *J Clin Onc.* 2011; 29:27, 3669–3676.

CHAPTER 6

Management of High-Risk Prostate Cancer—Adjuvant and Neoadjuvant Strategies

■ Introduction

■ In the previous chapter, it was shown that current surgical and radiotherapeutic techniques have the potential for curing a large percentage of clinically localized prostate cancers. Yet, many patients will experience relapse and go on to die of their disease despite the fact that their tumors appeared localized. This chapter reviews treatment options for patients at high risk of failure.

■ Definitions

■ High-risk prostate cancer
  * There is no clear-cut consensus as to what constitutes high risk of failure. Most clinicians would agree that the following pre-treatment clinical findings increase the risk of failure.
    ■ Clinical stage of T3 or higher
    ■ Combined Gleason score of 8–10
    ■ PSA level greater than 20 ng/ml
    ■ Multiple positive biopsy cores (> 3)
    ■ Extensive involvement of biopsy cores (> 50%)
  * Such factors alone or in combination may be less accurate than nomograms, which combine prognostic factors in a continuous manner.
    ■ Nomograms can be used to predict progression-free probabilities as well as pathologic stage.
    ■ This information can also be used in risk stratification for clinical trials.
      * For example, a neoadjuvant trial might choose a 5-year PFP of 70% or less by nomogram as being sufficiently high risk to justify eligibility.

- Clinicians therefore must examine high-risk prostate cancer trials reported in the literature with great care before generalizing conclusions. How was high risk defined? Were there sufficient numbers of patients from each high-risk category to justify the conclusions?

- Neoadjuvant therapy
  - Typically refers to systemic treatment administered before definitive surgery or radiotherapy
  - With the availability of more effective nonhormonal agents, chemotherapy and other drugs are now being studied in the neoadjuvant setting.
  - The goals of neoadjuvant treatment are to
    - Reduce the size of the primary tumor
    - Exert some control over occult micrometastatic disease in hopes of improving the cure rate
  - The major concerns about neoadjuvant therapy are
    - The relative inaccuracy of clinical staging
    - The possibility of tumor progression while definitive therapy is delayed
    - Neither of these is likely to be significant in prostate cancer.
      - Admittedly, DRE is notoriously inaccurate in assessing T stage. However, CT and more recently MRI (particularly with endorectal coil) offer the possibility of improved staging of the primary tumor and nearby structures such as the seminal vesicles, lymph nodes, and bones.
      - Prostate cancers are generally slow growing and virtually all of them respond to AST, reducing the likelihood of significant tumor progression while systemic therapy is being delivered.
    - High-risk prostate cancer is thus an ideal tumor in which to study neoadjuvant therapy.

- Adjuvant therapy
  - Refers to systemic treatment given after primary surgery because of adverse pathologic findings or after radiotherapy because pretreatment assessment suggests a high risk of recurrence

- High-risk pathological findings at surgery might include
  - Gleason scores (8–10)
  - Established extracapsular extension (T3a)
  - Seminal vesicle involvement (T3b)
  - Lymph node involvement (N1)
  - Positive surgical margins
  - Extension to nearby organs (T4)
- This chapter reviews combined modality therapy, focusing on high-risk disease.

■ Adjuvant/Neoadjuvant Strategies for Patients Undergoing Surgical Prostatectomy

- Neoadjuvant hormone therapy
- Neoadjuvant chemotherapy
- Adjuvant chemotherapy
- Adjuvant hormone therapy
- Adjuvant radiotherapy

■ Neoadjuvant Hormone Therapy Prior to Prostatectomy

- A number of trials, both randomized and nonrandomized, have addressed the issue of neoadjuvant AST prior to radical prostatectomy.[1] In most cases, the duration of AST prior to surgery was 3 months. The findings can be summarized as follows.
  - PSA values decreased in almost all patients. In one quarter to one-half of patients, the PSA levels became undetectable.
  - Neoadjuvant AST decreased the rate of positive surgical margins for small tumors (< T3) but not for larger tumors (≥ T3).
  - Neoadjuvant AST decreased the rate of extracapsular extension, thus increasing the likelihood of organ-confined disease.
  - Neoadjuvant AST had no effect on lymph node status or seminal vesicle involvement.
  - Periprostatic fibrosis caused by AST may make surgical dissection more difficult.
  - **No impact on relapse-free survival has been observed.**

■ Conclusion

 * Neoadjuvant AST cannot be considered standard therapy prior to radical prostatectomy. Whether or not a longer period of AST prior to surgery for patients with high-risk disease would be better is not known.

■ Neoadjuvant Chemotherapy Prior to Prostatectomy

■ With the availability of newer nonhormonal systemic therapies that demonstrate activity in advanced prostate cancer, the possibility of introducing them in the adjuvant or neoadjuvant setting becomes realistic. Despite the publication of several series, the question remains unsettled. Most of the reported studies are feasibility trials. The absence of randomized trials, the small numbers of patients entered, and the use of agents with marginal activity make it very difficult to draw conclusions. Further confounding the picture is the fact that several of the trials include hormone therapy.

■ The results of five trials of chemohormonal therapy and three trials of pure chemotherapy were summarized as of 2004.[2]

 * Common to all of these trials was the eligibility requirement of a high risk of treatment failure.
 * The number of patients entered into these trials ranged from 12–36.
 * None of the trials were randomized.
 * Follow-up was short.
 * Treatment regimens employed included
    ■ Chemohormonal neoadjuvant therapy
       * Ketoconazole and doxorubicin alternating with vinblastine and estramustine (both with combined androgen blockade [CAB])
       * Estramustine and etoposide
       * Paclitaxel plus carboplatin plus estramustine plus goserelin acetate
       * Estramustine plus docetaxel plus CAB
       * Docetaxel plus estramustine

- ▓ Pure neoadjuvant chemotherapy
  - • Weekly docetaxel (2 trials)[2]
  - • Weekly docetaxel + mitoxantrone
- • Several findings were common to all these studies.
  - ▓ Toxicity was generally acceptable.
    - • Thromboembolic events were noted in patients receiving estramustine.
  - ▓ Almost all patients had a decrease in PSA levels.
  - ▓ In up to 50% of patients, serum PSA levels became undetectable.
  - ▓ No pathologic complete responses were reported.
- ▓ A Cancer and Leukemia Group B (CALGB) trial (90203) is currently underway with a target of 700 high-risk patients identified as:
  - • A predicted 5-year, disease-free probability of < 60% by Kattan nomogram OR
  - • Any patient with Gleason score equal to or greater than 8
  - • All patients must be otherwise eligible for a radical prostatectomy.
  - • Any patient with Gleason 8 or higher
  - • Patients are randomly assigned to immediate prostatectomy versus six cycles of neoadjuvant docetaxel plus 12–24 weeks of androgen-suppressive therapy prior to prostatectomy.
- ▓ Conclusion
  - • Earlier studies establish the feasibility of neoadjuvant chemotherapy, but until the results of CALGB 90203 are available, the standard of care for high-risk patients undergoing surgery remains immediate prostatectomy.
  - • As of this writing, there is no high level evidence to justify the use of cytotoxic chemotherapy after surgery for high-risk disease.

■ Adjuvant Androgen-Suppressive Therapy after Prostatectomy

■ The use of androgen-suppressive therapy immediately after radical prostatectomy for high-risk disease was investigated in a randomized Eastern Cooperative Oncology Group (ECOG 3886) trial published by Messing et al.[3] in 1999 and updated in 2006.[4]

  • Men with positive lymph nodes were assigned to either immediate (continuous) androgen-suppressive therapy (goserelin or orchiectomy) or to androgen-suppressive therapy at the time of manifest progression.

  • 98 patients were evaluable, and median follow-up was 11.9 years. Early androgen-suppressive therapy showed advantages in:

    ■ Overall survival: 64% versus 45% hazard ratio (HR) 1.84 $p = 0.04$

    ■ Disease-specific survival: 85% vs 51% HR 4.09 $p = 0.0004$

    ■ Progression-free survival: 53% versus 14% HR 3.42 $p \leq 0.0001$

  • Although this study strongly supports the use of immediate androgen-suppressive therapy for node-positive disease, the lack of central pathology review and the limitation of AST in the delayed treatment arm for patients with manifest recurrence, failure has limited the acceptance of these results.

■ There are no randomized trials that examine the usefulness of adjuvant hormone therapy for other high-risk groups, such as those with established extracapsular extension, seminal vesicle involvement, or high Gleason scores.

■ A much larger European investigation examined the value of concurrent bicalutamide (150 mg/day) in addition to surgery, radiotherapy, or observation in a series of three randomized, double-blind studies.[5]

  • Preliminary results indicate improved (longer) time to relapse for the high-dose bicalutamide arm,[6] but the possibility of an increased overall death rate in that arm has been raised.[7]

- ▓ Conclusion
    - ● Based on the ECOG 3886, immediate AST should be considered for patients with positive nodes found at the time of prostatectomy. There is no evidence to support the use of immediate androgen suppression in node-negative patients who have other high-risk pathological features.

■ Adjuvant Radiotherapy after Prostatectomy

- ▓ Radiotherapy administered to patients with high-risk disease immediately after prostatectomy has been the subject of a number of nonrandomized trials.
- ▓ Two randomized trials were recently reported
    - ● EORTC 22911[8]
        - ▓ Patients undergoing radical retropubic prostatectomy were eligible if they had:
            - ● pT3a or pT3b N0 disease
            - ● Extracapsular extension
            - ● Positive surgical margins
            - ● Seminal vesicle involvement
            - ● No lymph node involvement
        - ▓ Eligible patients (1005) were randomized to receive immediate adjuvant radiotherapy or observation. Androgen-suppressive therapy was not administered.
        - ▓ Almost two-thirds of the patients had positive surgical margins.
        - ▓ One-quarter of the patients had seminal vesicle involvement.
        - ▓ Patients with detectable PSA postsurgery were not excluded.
        - ▓ Endpoints were biochemical progression-free survival and clinical progression-free survival
        - ▓ Results: With a follow up of 5 years:
            - ● Improved freedom from biochemical progression was observed for patients receiving adjuvant radiotherapy compared to those who were watched (74% vs. 52.6%, p = .0001).

- Clinical progression-free survival was better for patients receiving radiotherapy compared to those who were observed (14.9% vs. 22.5%, p = .0009).
- Patients receiving radiotherapy also had statistically significant less local recurrences at 5 years.
  - Re-analysis suggests that patients with positive surgical margins benefit most from adjuvant radiotherapy.
  - There was no difference in overall survival.
- The incidence of grade 3 bowel or urinary toxicity at 5 years was less than 5% and similar in both groups.
- SWOG 8794[9]
  - 425 patients with pT3a, pT3b, or positive surgical margins were randomized to immediate radiotherapy or observation. With a median follow up of > 12.5 years:
    - Adjuvant radiotherapy improved.
    - Overall survival
      - 15.3 years versus 13.3 years
      - HR 0.72
        - 95% confidence interval (CI) (0.55–0.96)
      - p = 0.023
    - Metastases-free survival
      - 14.7 versus 12.9 years
      - HR 0.71
        - 95% CI (0.54–0.94)
      - p = 0.016
  - *Note:* This is the only randomized trial showing a survival advantage for immediate adjuvant radiotherapy for prostatectomy patients with pT3 N0 disease.
- Many patients in the ECOG 22911 and SWOG 8794 had detectable PSA post-prostatectomy, leaving unanswered the question of radiotherapy in patients with undetectable PSA postsurgery, theoretically a more favorable subset.

- A German study attempts to address that issue.[10]
  - 385 men with pT3 N0 disease and undetectable postop PSA levels were randomized to immediate postoperative radiotherapy or observation.
  - Immediate radiotherapy improved biochemical relapse-free survival at 5 years.
    - 54% versus 72%
    - HR 0.53 with 95% CI4 of 0.37–0.79
    - p = 0.0015
- Taken together, these three studies offer evidence for the benefit of immediate radiotherapy to the prostate bed for patients with pT3–T4 disease or positive surgical margins but negative lymph nodes. However, only one of the studies (SWOG 8794) has shown a survival advantage.
- As such, adjuvant radiotherapy to begin after recovery from surgery should be considered for patients with pT3–T4 disease and those with positive surgical margins if they are lymph-node negative.
- The three studies do not address the issue of immediate radiotherapy versus radiotherapy at time of PSA failure nor do they address the role of androgen suppression for this subset of patients.
- As a result, not all clinicians recommend immediate radiotherapy for these patients.
- Some prefer waiting for PSA failure.[11]
  - The optimal management of very high risk patients pT3–T4 who are also node positive is not yet known.

■ Neoadjuvant/Adjuvant Strategies for Patients Undergoing Radiotherapy

- Neoadjuvant chemotherapy
- Neoadjuvant/adjuvant hormone therapy

■ Neoadjuvant Chemotherapy Prior to Radiotherapy

■ Two nonrandomized studies[12,13] have reported the feasibility of neoadjuvant chemotherapy prior to radiotherapy for high-risk disease. Concurrent androgen-suppressive therapy makes interpretation difficult. At this time, chemotherapy prior to radiotherapy remains experimental.

■ A trial currently underway will compare radiotherapy plus androgen suppression versus the same plus docetaxel prior to and during radiotherapy.

■ The use of neoadjuvant chemotherapy prior to or during radiotherapy is not supported by the evidence at this time.

■ Neoadjuvant or Adjuvant Hormone Therapy and Radiotherapy

■ The *potential* benefits of androgen-suppressive therapy either before, during, or after radiotherapy include:
  * Enhanced radiobiologic effect
  * Reduction in target volume
  * Decreased bowel and urinary toxicity
  * Control of micrometastatic disease
  * Improved local control
  * Improved survival
  * Avoidance of higher radiation doses

■ A number of randomized trials have addressed some, but not all, of these questions. These trials are difficult to interpret for a number of reasons.
  * Differing definitions of high risk and varying eligibility.
    ■ Some allowed patients with clinically positive nodes and others did not.
  * Several trials involved both neoadjuvant and adjuvant therapy.
  * Many trials used older radiotherapy techniques and lower radiotherapy doses.
  * Some of the trials date back to the pre-PSA era.
  * Follow-up times have been generally short.

- Neoadjuvant AST trials in which hormone therapy was started at least 2 months before EBRT
  - RTOG 86-10[14]
    - This randomized trial involved 456 patients with bulky (5 × 5 cm as determined by DRE) tumors without distant spread.
    - Patients with regional lymphadenopathy were *not* excluded.
    - Patients were randomized to radiotherapy alone or to radiotherapy plus goserelin and flutamide, starting 2 months before radiation and continuing during radiotherapy.
    - At 10 years radiotherapy plus androgen suppression compared to radiotherapy alone
      - Reduced disease-specific mortality
        - 23% versus 36% p = 0.01
      - Decreased distant metastases
        - 35% verus 47% p = 0.006
      - Improved disease-free survival
        - 11% verus 3% p < 0.0001
      - There was a trend toward improved survival which was not statistically significant.
      - No differences in fatal cardiac events were noted.
    - However, subset analysis revealed that there was no statistically significant difference between the two arms for those patients with high Gleason scores (> 7).
    - For patients with Gleason scores of 2–6, all end points were superior for the AST arm compared with the radiotherapy alone arm, including survival (70% vs 52%, p = .015).
    - *Comment:* RTOG 86-10 suggests an advantage for short-term AST prior to and during radiotherapy versus radiotherapy alone for those patients with large primary tumors and low Gleason scores. The use of DRE to determine eligibility, the inclusion of some patients with positive regional nodes and the lack of PSA data limit the applicability of these results.

- RTOG 92-02[15]
  - This study, involving more than 1,500 men, compared short-term with long-term AST.
  - Eligibility required a clinical stage of T2c or higher with a PSA level of less than 150 ng/ml.
  - All patients received goserelin and flutamide for 2 months before and 2 months during radiotherapy.
  - Patients assigned to the first arm received no further AST.
  - Patients assigned to the other arm received an additional 24 months of AST.
  - Long-term AST was associated with increased risk of late grade 3–4 gastrointestinal toxicity.

Table 6-1 Adjuvant Androgen Suppressive Therapy: Short Term vs. Long Term

End Point	LTAD	STAD	P Value
Disease-free survival, %	46.4	28.1	p ≤ .0001
bPFP, %	72.0	45.5	p ≤ .0001
Local control, %	93.6	87.7	p ≤ .0001
Overall survival (entire cohort), %	80.0	78.5	p = .73
Overall survival (Gleason score ≥ 8), %	81.0	70.7	p = .044

- Results
  - Long-term androgen suppression (LTAS) was significantly better than short-term (STAS) in the following end points:
    - Disease-free survival
    - Reduction in local recurrence
    - Reduction in distant metastases
    - Increased time to PSA failure
  - At 10 years, overall survival, however, was not significantly different except for patients with Gleason scores of 8–10. 31.9% vs 45.1% p = 0.0061

■ *Comment:* RTOG 9202 suggests a benefit for long-term AST plus radiotherapy over short-term AST for patients with high-grade advanced local tumors. The inclusion of a subset analysis that was not originally planned, and the inclusion of patients with very high PSA levels in both groups, detract from the conclusions drawn. Finally, this study does not really answer the question of neo-adjuvant AST benefits, as there was no control arm undergoing radiotherapy alone.

Adjuvant AST Trials in which Hormone Therapy was Started Concurrent with or after Institution of EBRT

■ Single-agent high-dose (150 mg/day) bicalutamide with radiotherapy is discussed earlier. Preliminary results indicate improved time to progression. Increased mortality in the bicalutamide arm is of concern.[7]

■ As discussed earlier, RTOG 92-02 suggested a benefit in overall survival for prolonged rather than short-term AST.

■ Pilepich et al.[16] (RTOG 85-31) randomized 977 patients to EBRT alone or to EBRT plus adjuvant goserelin, starting the last week of radiotherapy and continuing indefinitely.

  * Patients at high risk were identified as having clinical stage T3 or higher or regional lymph node involvement.

  * Patients at high risk after surgery, as defined by positive surgical margins or seminal vesicle involvement, were also eligible. However, it should be noted that only 15% of patients entered were in this category.

  * Patients with very bulky primary tumors were not eligible and were considered for a neoadjuvant trial (RTOG 86-10), unless they had nodal metastases outside the pelvis.

- Patients on the control arm were given goserelin at the time of progression. At 10 years, the following was observed:

Table 6-2 Immediate vs. Delayed Adjuvant Androgen Suppression With EBRT

End Point	Adjuvant ADT + EBRT	EBRT	P Value
Overall survival, %	49	39	p = .002
Local failure, %	23	38	p < .0001
Biochemical failure, %	69	91	p < .0001
Distant metastases, %	24	39	p < .001
Disease-specific mortality, %	16	22	p = .0052

- Those patients receiving immediate androgen-suppressive therapy had improved survival (49% vs 39%, p = 0.002).
- There was no survival advantage at 10 years for patients with Gleason scores of less than 7.
- *Comment:* This is a large truly adjuvant study, although it could be argued that RTOG 85-31 really compares immediate with delayed AST. Nonetheless, it appears to show a benefit for adjuvant AST in patients with high-stage, high-grade tumors. The very wide eligibility allowances make this a very mixed population. The small number of surgical patients makes it impossible to draw conclusions as to the benefit of immediate AST in the high-risk postsurgical setting. The improvement in overall survival for the entire cohort seems to be due to the effect on patients with high-grade disease.
- Bolla et al.[17] reported in 2002 and updated in 2010[18] the long-term follow-up of a European Organization for Research and Treatment of Cancer (EORTC 22863) study first published in 1997.
  - This trial randomized 415 patients to either EBRT alone or EBRT plus 3 years of AST with goserelin started at the time of irradiation. (Patients also received a month of cyproterone acetate, starting a few days before goserelin in order to prevent a testosterone flare reaction.)

- Eligibility criteria included clinical stage T3 or T4 N0 with any histologic grade, and T1 or T2 with high grade (WHO 3). The latter group comprised less than 10% of the cohort.
- With a median follow-up of 9.1 years, adjuvant AST + EBRT was superior to EBRT alone in:
  - 10-year clinical disease-free survival
    - 47.7% versus 22.7%, HR 0.42, p = 0.0001
  - 10-year overall survival
    - 58.1 % versus 39.8%, HR 0.60, p = 0.0004
  - 10-year prostate-specific mortality
    - 10.3% versus 30.4%, HR 0.38, p = 0.0001
      - Risk of locoregional progression
        - 6.0% versus 23.5%, HR 0.21, p < 0.0001

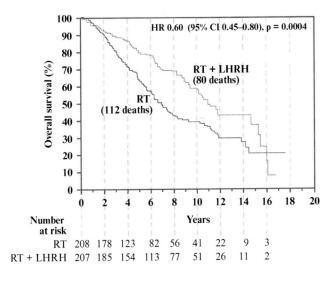

Figure 6-1 Kaplan-Meier estimates of overall survival by treatment group. O = number of deaths; N = number of patients. RT = radiotherapy. LHRH = luteinising-hormone-releasing hormone. Bolla M, van Tienhoven G, Warde P, et al. External irradiation with or without long-term androgen suppression for prostate cancer with high metastatic risk: ten year results of an EORTC randomized study. *Lancet Oncology.* 2010;11:1066–73.

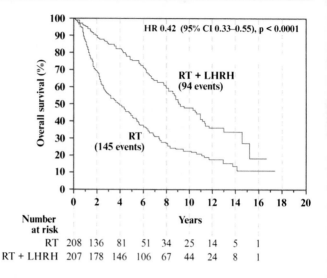

Figure 6-2 Kaplan-Meier estimates of the biochemically defined disease-free survival. O = number of failures; N = number of patients. Bolla M, van Tienhoven G, Warde P, et al. External irradiation with or without long-term androgen suppression for prostate cancer with high metastatic risk: ten year results of an EORTC randomized study. *Lancet Oncology.* 2010;11:1066–73.

- *Comment:* This study lends further support for the use of adjuvant AST in patients with locally advanced tumors. No conclusion can be drawn as to the benefit of adjuvant AST in patients who are at high risk by virtue of high tumor grade alone. The radiotherapy doses administered in this study would now be considered low by most radiation oncologists.

- D'Amico et al.[19] randomized 206 patients to receive either 70 Gy 3DCRT (to the prostate and seminal vesicles) alone or the same 3DCRT with 6 months of AST (gonadotropin-releasing hormone [GnRH] agonist plus flutamide).
  - Patients eligible for this trial were considered to be at high risk if they had Gleason scores of 7 or higher, a PSA level of between 10 and 40 ng/ml, or stage T3 disease by MRI with endorectal coil.

- Hormone therapy with a GnRH analog and flutamide was started 2 months before and continued during radiotherapy and for 2 months after, for a total of 6 months.
- At a median follow-up of 7.6 years, there was:
  - A significantly increased risk of all cause mortality (HR 1.8, 95% CI of 1.1–2.9, p = 0.01) for patients who received radiotherapy alone
  - The subset of patients without serious comorbidities seems to have had a more pronounced benefit. Men in this group who received radiotherapy alone had a much greater chance of dying than those who received radiotherapy and androgen-suppressive therapy (HR 4.2, 95% CI of 2.1–8.5, p < 0.001).
  - The presence of severe comorbidity seems to have erased the benefit, presumably due to death from unrelated causes.
- *Comment:* It is important to note that this study used 3DCRT techniques as opposed to the other trials in which older radiation techniques were employed. It showed that short-term AST therapy seemed to benefit high-risk patients with disease, although the use of salvage AST in patients who experienced treatment failure may have diminished the actual effect.
- EORTC 22961 is another study supporting longer versus shorter periods of androgen-suppressive therapy with radiotherapy for high-risk patients.[20]
  - 970 patients with T1c–T2b N1–N2 or T2–T4 N0–N2
  - Patients had to be M0 and have a PSA < 40 times the upper limit of normal.
- At 6.4 years of follow-up, overall mortality was decreased for patients receiving long-term androgen-suppressive therapy.
  - 15% versus 19% 5-year mortality (HR 1.42, 95% CI of 1.09–1.85)
  - This trial attempted to show non-inferiority of short-term AST compared to long-term AST, but failed, indicating that short-term AST was inferior.

* The use of androgen-suppressive therapy with transperineal seed implants is not addressed by clinical trials at this time. One reason may be that the kind of high-risk patients who have been enrolled in the clinical trials cited here, are more likely to receive EBRT.
* Neoadjuvant or adjuvant androgen-suppressive therapy is commonly used in men who have very large prostate glands prior to either EBRT or seed implants regardless of risk categorization in order to reduce prostate size hoping to lessen toxicity. This practice is not based on strong evidence from clinical trials.

■ Summary and Conclusions on High-Risk Prostate Cancer

* Radical retropubic prostatectomy can be considered (in addition to EBRT) for young, healthy men with high-risk disease.
* There is no established role for neoadjuvant AST or chemotherapy prior to surgery for high-risk patients except as part of a clinical trial.
* Patients who are found to have positive lymph nodes at the time of surgery should be considered for AST based on EORTC 3886.
* The role for adjuvant AST is not established for other high-risk situations after surgery, such as extracapsular extension, positive surgical margins, or seminal vesicle involvement.
* There is no proven role for the routine use of chemotherapy after radical prostatectomy.
* Adjuvant radiotherapy should be considered for patients with pT3 a or b or disease or positive surgical margins at surgery who are node negative (SWOG 8794). The management of patients with pT3a, pT3b, or those with positive surgical margins AND positive nodes is not defined, since the presence of positive nodes at surgery excluded patients from those clinical trials.

- The preponderance of evidence gathered from a number of clinical trials cited earlier supports the use of androgen-suppressive therapy in conjunction with external-beam radiotherapy for high-risk and maybe intermediate-risk patients.
  - Several factors make these the results of these trials confusing for clinicians attempting to integrate these findings into clinical practice
    - Wide variation in risk assessment
      - Most are based on clinical staging
      - PSA eligibility varied
      - Gleason scores not commonly used
    - Radiotherapy techniques tended to be older
    - Radiotherapy doses tended to be lower than are commonly used now
    - Variation in timing of start of androgen suppression with respect to the start of radiotherapy
  - Some trends can be discerned
    - Androgen suppressive therapy is probably not needed for patients undergoing external beam radiotherapy for low-risk prostate cancer
    - Longer courses (36 months) of androgen suppression seem superior to shorter courses (4–6 months) for high-risk patients.
    - Shorter courses (4–6 months) of therapy may be sufficient for those with intermediate-risk disease
    - Although androgen supressive therapy was started prior to radiotherapy in some studies, it remains unclear whether or not neoadjuvant treatment is needed.
    - In all the studies, androgen suppressive therapy was underway during radiotherapy
    - Most studies cited above used combined androgen blockade
      - The role of monotherapy with an LHRH agonist is not defined.
- Whether or not the benefits of androgen suppression pertain to patients treated in the new era of high-dose, intensity-modulated, and image-guided radiotherapy is not known.

- There is no role for either adjuvant or neoadjuvant chemotherapy for patients undergoing any form of radiotherapy.
- *Comment:* Once again, these are recommendations and should not be interpreted as strict guidelines. Allowance must be made for clinical judgment and individual circumstances. Clinicians dealing with high-risk patients should follow the literature carefully as important clinical trials addressing these questions mature and become available for scrutiny. The availability of effective new systemic therapies such as abiraterone acetate and MDV 3100 will in all probability lead to a number of new adjuvant trials.

■ References

1. Wieder J, Soloway MS. Neoadjuvant androgen deprivation before radical prostatectomy for prostate adenocarcinoma. In: Kantoff PW, Carroll PR, D'Amico AV, eds. *Prostate Cancer: Principles and Practice.* Philadelphia: Lippincott Williams and Wilkins; 2002;431–443.
2. Alumkal J, Carducci MA. Early use of chemotherapy in conjunction with radical prostatectomy. *Clin Prostate Cancer.* 2004;3:144–149.
3. Messing EM, Manola J, Sarosdy M, Wilding G, Crawford ED, Trump D. Immediate hormonal therapy compared with observation after radical prostatectomy and pelvic lymphadenectomy in men with node-positive prostate cancer. *N Engl J Med.* 1999;341:1781–1788.
4. Messing EM, Manola J, Yao J, Kiernan M, Crawford D, Wilding G, di'SantAgnese PA, Trump D; Immediate versus deferred androgen deprivation treatment in patients with node-positive prostate cancer after radical prostatectomy and pelvic lymphadenectomy. Eastern Cooperative Oncology Group study EST 3886. *Lancet Oncology.* 2006; 7 (6):472–479.
5. See WA, McLeod D, Iversen P, Wirth M. The bicalutamide Early Prostate Cancer Program. Demography. *Urol Oncol.* 2001;6:43–47.
6. See WA. Adjuvant hormone therapy after radiation or surgery for localized or locally advanced prostate cancer. *Curr Treat Options Oncol.* 2003;4:351–362.

7. See WA, Wirth MP, McLeod DG, et al. Bicalutamide as immediate therapy either alone or as adjuvant to standard care of patients with localized or locally advanced prostate cancer: first analysis of the early prostate cancer program. *J Urol.* 2002;168:429–435.

8. Bolla M, van Poppel H, Collette L, Vekemans K, Da Pozzo L, de Reijke T, et al. Postoperative radiotherapy after radical prostatectomy: a randomized controlled trial (EORTC trial 22911). *Lancet.* 2005;366:572–578.

9. Thompson IM, Tangen Cm, Paradelo J, et al. Adjuvant radiotherapy for pathological T3N0M) prostate cancer reduces risk of metastases and improves survival: long term followup of a randomized clinical trial. *J. Urol.* 2009;181: 956–962.

10. Wiegel T, Bottke D, Steiner U, et al. Phase III Postoperative Adjuvant Radiotherapy After Radical Prostatectomy Compared With Radical Prostatectomy Alone in pT3 Prostate Cancer With Postoperative Undetectable Prostate-Specific Antigen: ARO 96-02/AUO AP 09/95. *J Clin Onc.* 2009;18 (27): 2924–2930.

11. Ward JF, Blute ML. Use and timing of radiotherapy in high-risk prostate cancer. *JAMA.* 2004;291:2817.

12. Ryan CJ, Zelefsky MJ, Heller G, et al. Five-year outcomes after neoadjuvant chemotherapy and conformal radiotherapy in patients with high-risk localized prostate cancer. *Urology.* 2004;64:90–94.

13. Ben-Josef E, Porter AT, Hans S, et al. Neoadjuvant estramustine and etoposide followed by concurrent estramustine and definitive radiotherapy for locally advanced prostate cancer: feasibility and preliminary results. *Int J Radiat Oncol Biol Phys.* 2001;49:699–703.

14. Roach M, Bae K, Speicht J, et al. Short-term neoadjuvant androgen deprivation therapy and external-beam radiotherapy for locally advanced prostate cancer: long-term results of RTOG 8610. *J Clin Oncol.* 2008;26(4):585–591.

15. Horwitz EM, Bae K, Pilepich M et al. Ten year follow-up of radiation therapy oncology group protocol 92-02: a phase III trial of the duration of elective androgen deprivation in locally advance prostate cancer. *J Clin Oncol.* 2008; 26(15):2497–504.

16. Pilepich MV, Winter K, Lawton CA, et al. Androgen suppression adjuvant to definitive radiotherapy in prostate carcinoma—long-term results of phase III RTOG 85-31. *Int J Radiat Oncol Biol Phys.* 2005;61:1285–1290.

17. Bolla M, Collette L, Blank L, et al. Long-term results with immediate androgen suppression and external irradiation in patients with locally advanced prostate cancer (an EORTC study): a phase III randomised trial. *Lancet.* 2002;360:103–106.

18. Bolla M, Van Tienhoven G, Warde P, Dubois JB, Mirimanoff RO, Storme G, Bernier J, Kuten A, Sternberg C, Billiet I, Torecilla JL, Pfeffer R, Cutajar CL, Van der Kwast T, Collette L. External irradiation with or without long-term androgen suppression for prostate cancer with high metastatic risk: 10-year results of an EORTC randomised study. *Lancet Oncology.* 2010;11(11):1066–1073.

19. D'Amico AV, Chen MH, Renshaw AA, et al. Androgen suppression and radiation vs. radiation alone for prostate cancer. *JAMA.* 2008;299:289–295.

20. Bolla, M, de Reijke TM and van Tienhoven G. Duration of androgen suppression in the treatment of prostate cancer. *N Engl J Medicine.* 2009;24 (360): 2516–2527.

Section IV
Clinical State:
Rising PSA

CHAPTER 7

Biochemical Failure and Salvage Therapy

■ Biochemical Failure

Introduction

An increase in the level of PSA is usually the first sign that a patient has experienced relapse after primary surgical or radiotherapeutic treatment of his prostate cancer. After radical prostatectomy, the PSA level should decline to undetectable amounts within 6 weeks. After radiotherapy (EBRT or seed implantation) the PSA levels may fluctuate for 1–2 years or even longer before reaching nadir. Although the definition of biochemical (or PSA) failure varies, most agree that a sustained increase in PSA levels indicates persistent or recurrent disease. The availability and pervasive use of this marker results in a large cohort of men who feel well, but suffer from the knowledge that their disease has not been cured. The pressure brought to bear on the physician to "do something" can be significant.

Because men with prostate cancer can remain asymptomatic and without manifest evidence of their disease for many years after biochemical failure,[1] management decisions are complicated. If curative options exist, few would withhold them. But, in practicality, it may be very difficult to distinguish between those patients with purely local recurrence who might enjoy a long-term, disease-free remission (or cure) with further local therapy from those with distant spread, for whom any therapy would be palliative. This chapter discusses the natural history of biochemical failure and the therapeutic options available to men in this situation.

- Definition of biochemical failure[2]
  - After surgery
    - The serum PSA level should drop to less than 0.1 ng/ml using routine testing and less than 0.05 ng/ml when the supersensitive assay is used.
    - The PSA should be undetectable by 6–8 weeks after surgery.
      - The Johns Hopkins Group defines PSA failure at a level of 0.2 ng/ml or higher by standard measurements.
    - Although the entire prostate is removed in the course of a prostatectomy, the possibility of residual benign prostatic tissue should be considered when biochemical levels become detectable by supersensitive techniques but are extremely low (< 0.1 ng/ml).
    - That being the case, it would be prudent to observe a sustained and increasing rise in biochemical levels (as per the definition described later) before diagnosing biochemical failure. On the other hand, the biochemical level at which failure is defined should not be so high that it exceeds the threshold for salvage radiation (see Salvage Radiotherapy).
  - After radiation
    - The biochemical nadir may not be reached for 1–2 years.
    - PSA levels may fluctuate secondary to a "bounce" effect after radiation.
    - Low levels of PSA due to residual benign prostate tissue may persist.
    - Biochemical failure after radiation, as defined by American Society of Therapeutic Radiology and Oncology (ASTRO), is any increase of at least 2.0 ng/mL above nadir.[3]
- Natural history of biochemical failure after radical prostatectomy
  - The updated data from Johns Hopkins[4] provide useful information about the natural course of this entity in the postsurgical setting.

- This was a retrospective study involving 3,263 patients who underwent radical prostatectomy and no adjuvant therapy.
  - 10% developed biochemical failure.
  - With median follow-up of 10.5 years, 44% of those who experienced biochemical failure developed metastases.
  - Median actuarial time from biochemical failure to metastases was 7 years.
  - Factors that predicted increased risk of metastases over time were
    - High Gleason score (8–10)
    - Biochemical failure within 2 years of surgery
    - Biochemical doubling time of less than 10 months
  - Biochemical doubling time was also shown to be predictive of metastases and cancer-specific mortality after radiation.[5]
- Imaging the patient with biochemical failure
  - Reasons to image patients with biochemical failure include
    - To clarify patient symptoms, abnormal laboratory values (other than biochemical), or physical examination findings
    - To determine whether distant metastases are present
    - To distinguish between purely local recurrence and distant metastases in order to identify patients who might benefit from salvage therapy
  - As always in medicine, the clinician should always ask the question, "What am I going to do differently based on the results of these studies?"
    - For example, the distinction between local and distant relapse becomes moot if the patient is not a candidate for potentially curative salvage therapy because, for example, of advanced age or severe co-morbidities.
    - Some patients, and their physicians, may choose to continue observation even in the presence of small-volume clinically manifest but asymptomatic metastases.

- Further complicating the issue is the fact that the effects of prior treatment and the low tumor burden usually associated with biochemical relapse reduces both sensitivity and selectivity of current imaging techniques.
- Suggested guidelines for imaging patients with biochemical failure
  - Once again, these are suggestions rather than firm guidelines, as evidence-based data are sparse.
  - Appropriate imaging is indicated when symptoms, an abnormal physical examination, or abnormal laboratory studies need clarification.
  - Imaging should be considered if the PSA level is greater than 10 ng/ml or if the PSA level is rapidly doubling.
    - The threshold for imaging should be lower in patients with high-grade, undifferentiated, or neuroendocrine tumors.
  - Imaging should be considered when a palpable abnormality is found in the prostate fossa. In that case, MRI of the prostate (with endorectal coil when available) is the technique of choice.
  - Imaging should be done before a patient is referred for salvage prostatectomy, salvage radiotherapy, or a clinical trial.
  - Baseline scans should be obtained before instituting AST.
- Imaging techniques[6]
  - CT of the abdomen and pelvis
    - May be useful to evaluate
      - The prostate or prostate fossa and nearby structures
      - Lymph nodes
      - Soft tissue
      - Viscera
      - Bones
    - Demonstrates very low yield at very low PSA levels

- Radionuclide (technetium Tc 99m diphosphonate) bone scan
  - Safe, inexpensive study
  - Many benign conditions can cause false-positives
  - True-positives unlikely when PSA level is very low[6]
- MRI
  - Excellent visualization of the prostate gland or prostatic bed
  - Superior to CT in detecting local recurrence, particularly when used with endorectal coil
  - Allows evaluation of nearby nodes and bony structures
  - May be useful, particularly in clarifying ambiguous findings on bone scan
  - Regional lymph node–bearing areas can be evaluated, but CT preferable for abdominal (retroperitoneal) nodes
  - Value of high resolution MRI with superparamagnetic iron oxide nanoparticles remains unproven at this time (see Chapter 4, Staging and Risk Assessment)
  - Indium In 111 capromab pendetide (ProstaScint) (see Chapter 4, Staging and Risk Assessment)
    - Interpretation difficult because of poor image quality
    - High false-positive and false-negative rates[7]
    - Suggestion of better long-term biochemical failure control with salvage radiotherapy when this study is negative for distant metastases[8] not confirmed in other trials[9]
    - Usefulness in detecting local recurrence or nodal metastases remains unclear
  - Fluorodeoxyglucose (FDG)-PET
    - Excretion by the kidneys and consequent accumulation in the bladder limits the usefulness of this technique in evaluating prostate bed recurrence.
    - Hormone-sensitive prostate cancer may not be hypermetabolic by FDG-PET.

- Newer labels that are not renally excreted, such as choline and acetate, show promise for diagnosing local recurrence.
- Using dihydrotestosterone rather than glucose may allow more specific targeting of prostate cancer cells.
- FDG-PET may be more useful in identifying distant sites in the castrate-resistant state
  - *Comment:* Imaging the patient with biochemical failure remains problematic. At the low PSA levels at which imaging is usually triggered, current techniques do not satisfactorily locate the site of recurrence or distinguish between local and distant disease. In the absence of convincing imaging results, management decisions are made on clinical grounds.
- The clinical distinction between local and systemic failure
  - Factors favoring systemic recurrence
    - High initial Gleason score (8–10)
    - Very high PSA levels at presentation (> 20)
    - Seminal vesicle or lymph node involvement at surgery
    - Failure to reach expected PSA nadir after primary therapy
    - Short (< 12 months) interval between primary therapy and biochemical failure
    - Short PSA doubling time[10]
  - Factors favoring isolated local recurrence
    - Low to intermediate Gleason score
    - Low PSA levels at presentation
    - Absence of seminal vesicle or lymph node involvement at surgery
    - Positive surgical margins at surgery
    - Long interval between primary therapy and biochemical relapse
    - Longer PSA doubling time[10]

Table 7-1 Patterns of Recurrence after Radical Prostatectomy[11]

Variable	Local Recurrence	Distant Metastases ± Local Recurrence
Number of patients, no. (%)	41 (34)	88 (66)
Gleason score, %		
2–4	0	0
5–6	55	45
7	39	61
8–10	11	89
Pathologic stage, %		
Organ-confined	40	60
Capsular penetration, negative surgical margins	54	46
Capsular penetration, positive surgical margins	48	52
Seminal vesicle involvement	16	84
Lymph node metastases	7	93
Timing of PSA recurrence, %		
Within 1 year	7	93
Within 1–2 years	10	90
After year 2	61	39
After year 3	74	26

Data from Pound CR, Partin AW, Epstein JI, Walsh PC. Prostate-specific antigen after anatomic radical retropubic prostatectomy. Patterns of recurrence and cancer control. *Urol Clin North Am*. 1997;24:395–406.

- *Comment:* Given the widespread and frequent use of the PSA test, starting shortly after primary therapy, most men with biochemical failure are diagnosed when their PSA levels are very low. Imaging at that time is rarely helpful, requiring decisions to be made based on clinical criteria. The end result is that uncertainty about the precise location(s) of the recurrence is very common. For patients who are not candidates for salvage therapy, the issue becomes moot, and the only choice becomes one of whether to institute immediate palliative hormone therapy or to continue observation. On the other hand, absent compelling evidence of distant spread, strong consideration should be given to salvage therapy depending on the overall status of the patient and the clinical circumstances.

- Options for managing patients with biochemical failure
  - Noncurative options
    - Observation
      - Main advantage is preservation of quality of life
      - May allow years without toxicity from treatment or symptoms of disease[1]
        - Avoids loss of libido, hot flashes, osteoporosis, and other side effects of AST
      - Main disadvantage is anxiety over rising PSA levels
      - Attractive option for
        - The extreme elderly
        - Those with serious medical comorbidities that limit life expectancy
        - Men with long PSA doubling times[12]
        - Men who wish to preserve sexual function
      - The fact that observation is noncurative and that the patient's cancer will inevitably progress (unless he dies of something else) must be made clear to the patient and his family.
    - AST (see Chapter 8 for details)
      - This would include the following options:
        - Combined androgen blockade (CAB)
        - Luteinizing hormone-releasing hormone (LHRH) analog alone
        - Monotherapy with an antiandrogen
        - Surgical castration
        - Antiandrogen plus 5-alpha-reductase inhibitor (finasteride or dutasteride)
        - Intermittent androgen suppression
      - Can be used in patients after prostatectomy, radiotherapy, or both
      - May delay onset of clinically manifest metastases

- The impact on survival is modest in this setting[2]
- No randomized trials comparing AST with an observation arm in this setting
- Toxicity: see Chapter 8
- *Comment:* Extrapolation from trials discussed in Chapter 8 suggests a very modest benefit for early versus delayed AST, at least for some subsets of patients. Yet, the optimal timing for the institution of AST in patients with pure biochemical failure remains undetermined. Some clinicians base the decision to start AST on an arbitrary PSA level of > 10 or 20 ng/mL. Others will trigger treatment based on PSA-doubling time. The presence of symptomatic recurrent or metastatic disease is an indication to start systemic therapy in most patients. Most clinicians would agree that finding a significant volume of metastatic disease on imaging would also be an indication to start treatment, even if the patient has no symptoms. But, one could also argue that patients with asymptomatic small volume metastatic disease could be observed, and the author has seen patients who make that choice.
- Potentially curative options
  - Salvage radiotherapy
    - Salvage radiotherapy to the prostate bed for patients experiencing biochemical failure after radical prostatectomy offers the "only reasonable well-documented approach with curative potential."[2]
    - Durable biochemical freedom from progression rates vary between 25% and 50%.
      - Adverse factors (predictors of progression of disease):
        - Gleason score of 8–10
        - Preradiation PSA level greater than 2 ng/ml
        - Negative surgical margins
        - PSA doubling time of 10 months or shorter
        - Seminal vesicle involvement

- A large retrospective review involving more than 500 patients from 5 different tertiary referral centers was published in 2004.[13] In 2007 the study was expanded to include 1540 patients from 17 centers.[14]
- Patient characteristics
  - 1540 patients with biochemical failure after prostatectomy
  - Biochemical failure defined as PSA level of 0.2 ng/ml or greater at least 6 weeks after radical prostatectomy followed by another higher value or an absolute single PSA value of 0.5 ng/mL or higher
  - Patients who received adjunctive or concurrent androgen-suppressive therapy were excluded.
- Results (median follow-up: 45 months)
  - The 6-year overall PFP was 32% (95% CI of 28%–35%)
  - PFP varied with pretherapy PSA
    - 48% if PSA ≤ 0.5 ng/mL (95% CI of 40%–60%)
    - 40% if PSA is 0.51–1.00 ng/mL (95% CI of 34%–46%)
    - 28% if PSA is 1.01–1.5 ng/mL (95% CI of 20%–30%)
    - 18% if PSA > 1.50 ng/mL (95% CI of 14%–22%)
  - Even some subsets of patients with high-risk disease benefitted from salvage radiotherapy
    - 6-year PFP for patients with Gleason score > 8 or PSA-doubling time less than 10 months was 48% (95% CI of 35%–62%) if they had positive surgical margins and salvage radiotherapy was started when the PSA was less than or equal to 0.5ng/mL
  - A predictive nomogram based on these data was published in the 2007 paper.
- Toxicity
  - The majority had "mild to moderate" acute rectal and genitourinary toxicity.

- Although toxicity was not described in this report, data from other reports indicate a less than 10% rate of late urinary or rectal toxicity greater than grade 2.[10]
- Anecdotally, urinary incontinence does not seem to be increased by salvage radiotherapy.
- The impact of salvage radiotherapy on erectile function is not known but based on the experience with primary radiotherapy, some decline in erectile function can be expected.
  - *Comment:* Salvage radiotherapy is a reasonable and well-tolerated approach for patients with biochemical relapse after prostatectomy when the evidence points to local recurrence alone.
  - Current ASTRO recommendations suggest that radiotherapy should be started before the PSA level is greater than 1.5 ng/ml.[15]
    - Others have suggested even lower PSA level thresholds.
  - There is no role for "salvage" radiotherapy to the prostate bed in the presence of distant metastases, except perhaps in patients with very high-grade, undifferentiated tumors forming large, obstructing, or potentially obstructing, local prostate masses. In that case, radiotherapy would be palliative, not curative.
- Salvage radiotherapy and hormone therapy
  - Beyond in vitro data suggesting synergy between radiotherapy and AST, there are no evidence-based data to support the use of AST with radiotherapy in the salvage setting.
  - Trock[15] retrospectively reviewed 635 men with biochemical failure or local recurrence after radical prostatectomy who received salvage radiotherapy alone, salvage radiotherapy plus androgen suppression or observation. At median of 6 years after recurrence:
    - No salvage radiotherapy—22% died
    - Salvage radiotherapy alone—11% died
    - Salvage radiotherapy plus androgen suppression—12% died

- Men who received treatment more than 2 years after recurrence did not seem to benefit (in terms of prostate cancer–specific survival) from salvage radiotherapy.
- There was no benefit from the addition of androgen–suppressive therapy.
- Surprisingly, and in contradistinction to other studies, prostate-specific survival improvement was limited to those with rapid doubling times (< 6 months), independent of other factors.
- In this study, men whose PSA did not become undetectable did not enjoy improvement in prostate cancer-specific survival.

- Androgen suppression plus salvage radiotherapy
  - A prospective randomized controlled study comparing salvage radiotherapy alone versus salvage radiotherapy plus androgen suppression is currently underway (RTOG 0534).
    - This study also seeks to determine if radiotherapy to regional lymph nodes is needed in addition to radiotherapy to the prostate bed.
  - In clinical practice at many institutions, androgen suppressive therapy is given in conjunction with salvage radiotherapy based on extrapolation from studies done in the primary radiotherapy setting. The use of AST with salvage radiotherapy remains an issue of clinical judgment pending the results of pertinent clincial trials.
- Chemotherapy
  - Despite the availability of many new systemic therapy options for patients with advanced prostate cancer (see Chapter 9), there is no evidence that chemotherapy benefits patients with biochemical failure after primary therapy.
  - The Tax 3503 study, currently accruing patients who have biochemical failure after radical prostatectomy, randomly assigns subjects to androgen-suppressive therapy alone versus androgen-suppressive therapy plus docetaxel. The results of this trial are eagerly awaited.

- Salvage prostatectomy
  - Options are more limited for patients experiencing biochemical failure after radiotherapy. Although the addition of further radiotherapy by various means is being explored, these techniques are unproven and toxicity may be expected. Hormonal therapy, as described earlier, is a reasonable but noncurative option, as is observation.
  - Surgery is more difficult in an irradiated (or previously operated upon) pelvis, and thus the risk of complications is higher. Yet, for younger and otherwise healthy patients with a biopsy-proven local recurrence after radiotherapy, the risks may be acceptable in the absence of other potentially curative options.
  - In 2005 Ward et al.[17] reported more than 30 years of experience with salvage prostatectomy.
    - In this series, 199 patients underwent either salvage prostatectomy or salvage cystoprostatectomy.
    - All had biopsy-proven local recurrence indicating a significant tumor burden.
    - Surgical complication rates were low.
    - Continence (defined as needing 0 pads) was preserved in 50% of patients. Data were analyzed by type of procedure (radical prostatectomy alone vs radical cystoprostatectomy).
    - Results:

Table 7-2 Results of Salvage Prostatectomy and Salvage Cystoprostatectomy

	Overall	RP alone	CP
PFS, years	7.8	8.7	4.4
10-year cancer-specific survival, %	65	77	38

  - Potency
    - No data regarding potency were included in this report.
    - Other studies report 100% erectile dysfunction rates.[2]

- Stephenson and Eastham[18] reviewed their experience with salvage prostatectomy
  - 5-year progression-free probability ranged from 86%, for patients whose preoperative biochemical values were < 4 ng/ml, to 28% for patients with preoperative PSA values > 10 ng/ml.
  - When patients who underwent preradiotherapy lymph node dissections, or open (as opposed to transperineal) seed implants were excluded, preservation of continence was 68% in the patients who underwent salvage surgery after 1993.
  - Rectal injury in that same subset of patients was rare, 2–3%.
  - Anastamotic stricture rates were 17–32%.
  - Although data regarding potency were not included, cavernous nerve preservation was feasible such that selected patients may recover potency.
  - The author's opinion was that improved freedom from progression is possible when salvage prostatectomy is done earlier rather than later. Long-term freedom from progression was also noted to be related to the pathologic surgical stage.
- *Comment:* Salvage prostatectomy may have a role in select patients with biochemical failure. Continence and preservation of erectile function remain serious concerns for men considering this option. Because of the complexity and potential risks of this procedure, men being considered for it should have full preoperative medical evaluation.
- Newer approaches to patients with biochemical failure
  - A number of new approaches to the management of biochemical failure are under investigation. As of this writing, the proper role for these techniques has not been defined. They include:
    - Salvage external-beam radiotherapy after brachytherapy

- Salvage brachytherapy after EBRT
  * 50% 5-year freedom from progression rate reported.[19]
  * Better results may be expected with more careful case selection.
  * Toxicity not yet well characterized
- Salvage brachytherapy after prostatectomy
- Salvage cryotherapy
  * Potentially useful in both the postsurgical and postradiation settings
  * Although early cryotherapy techniques resulted in significant urinary toxicity, newer methods show more promise.[20]
- Chemotherapy with or without AST
  * The development of active agents for prostate cancer raises interest in using them in this setting.
  * Clinical trials are currently under way. Until they are completed, the use of chemotherapy for biochemical failure outside the setting of a clinical trial remains experimental.

■ Summary and Conclusions, Biochemical Relapse

- Patients with biochemical failure after primary therapy may do well, with no symptoms of their disease or toxicity from treatment for long periods of time.
- Imaging done to locate the site of recurrence and distinguish between local recurrence only and distant spread is generally not helpful unless the PSA level is very high or the patient's tumor is very undifferentiated.
- The distinction between local recurrence only and systemic disease is, by necessity, often based on clinical findings.
  * Absent compelling evidence of metastatic disease, patients with biochemical failure after primary prostatectomy should be considered for salvage radiotherapy and those with proven local recurrence after primary radiotherapy should be considered for salvage prostatectomy depending on their overall medical status and risk profile. These are the only potentially curative

modalities for biochemical failure after primary therapy. The decision to offer salvage therapy has to be weighed against the fact that many of these men may die of competing morbidities before they become symptomatic with recurrent prostate cancer.

- Watchful waiting, clearly a noncurative approach, is particularly worth considering in:
  - Patients who are not candidates for either salvage radiotherapy or surgery
  - Patients with severe medical comorbidities and those of very advanced age
  - Patients who prefer preserving sexual function
- AST may be considered in:
  - Patients who are not candidates for salvage radiotherapy or surgery and who are not comfortable with watchful waiting
    - The very modest advantage of starting AST in this setting and the risks associated with it (see Chapter 8) should be emphasized to the patient.
    - And, in the opinion of the author, androgen-suppressive therapy should be discouraged in patients whose only sign of relapse is PSA failure.
  - Patients with overt metastatic disease
  - Patients whose clinical findings suggest systemic rather than local recurrence
- Clinical trials to define the best treatment for biochemical failure are needed. The use of vaccines, antiangiogenic approaches, or targeted approaches in this low tumor-burden setting seems worthy of investigation.
- Finally and most important, there is no accepted standard treatment for patients with biochemical failure after surgery or radiotherapy.

■ Management of Overt Local Recurrence

- Salvage therapy is an ambiguous term. Most often, it refers to the attempt to cure patients whose only manifestation of recurrence is biochemical.
- Patients with a clinically detectable or biopsy-proven local recurrence after surgery or radiotherapy present a different

problem. In the absence of overt metastatic disease, patients with local recurrence may still be curable, but cure is probably less likely because of prior treatment and a larger tumor burden.

* Patients with large or bulky recurrences, particularly those with rectal or urinary tract obstruction, are not likely to be cured by surgery or radiotherapy.
* Palliative androgen-suppressive therapy should be instituted if the patient is noncastrate.
* Chemotherapy should be considered in patients whose tumors are castrate resistant.
* The role of radiotherapy in this setting is not well established but might be considered in patients who have dramatic reduction in the size of their tumors in response to systemic therapy and who have not received maximally tolerated radiotherapy doses.
* Salvage surgery, which might include pelvic exenteration, can be considered in the rare patient who is otherwise young and healthy and is willing to tolerate the considerable risks of such a procedure.
* Cryosurgery, high frequency ultrasound, and laser ablation should be discouraged in patients with very large, bulky prostatic tumors.
* Palliative colostomy or rectal stents may be needed for patients with complete rectal obstruction.
* Foley catheters, internal ureteral stents, or percutaneous nephrostomy may be needed for those with urinary tract obstruction.

▪ Patients with smaller localized recurrence and no evidence of metastases can be treated with:
  * Radiotherapy with or without androgen suppression
  * Androgen suppression alone
  * Surgery (select cases)
  * Cryosurgery

▪ In summary, patients with an isolated local recurrence after radiotherapy or surgery may be offered a variety of treatment options. There is very little data from clinical trials that might allow us to distinguish among them.

■ References

1. Pound CR, Partin AW, Eisenberger MA, Chan DW, Pearson JD, Walsh PC. Natural history of progression after biochemical elevation following radical prostatectomy. *JAMA*. 1999; 281:1591–1597.

2. Rosenbaum E, Partin AW, Eisenberger M. Biochemical relapse after primary treatment for prostate cancer: studies on natural history and therapeutic considerations. *JNCCN*. 2004;2:249–256.

3. American Society for Therapeutic Radiology and Oncology Consensus Panel. Consensus statement: guidelines for PSA following radiation therapy. *Int J Radiat Oncol Biol Phys*. 1997;37:1035–1041.

4. Eisenberger M, Partin AW, Pound CR, Roostelaar CV, Epstein J, Walsh PC. Natural history of progression of patients with biochemical (PSA) relapse following radical prostatectomy [abstract]. *Proc Am Soc Clin Oncol*. 2003; 22:380. Abstract 1527.

5. D'Amico AV, Moul J, Carroll PR, Sun L, Lubeck D, Chen MH. Cancer-specific mortality after surgery or radiation for patients with clinically localized prostate cancer managed during the prostate-specific antigen era. *J Clin Oncol*. 2003;21:2163–2172.

6. Hricak H, Schoder H, Pucar D, et al. Advances in imaging in the postoperative patient with a rising prostate-specific antigen level. *Semin Oncol*. 2003;30:616–634.

7. Kahn D, Williams RD, Seldin DW, et al. Radioimmuno-scintigraphy with 111 indium labeled CYT-356 for the detection of occult prostate cancer recurrence. *J Urol*. 1994; 152:1490–1495.

8. Kahn D, Williams RD, Haseman MK, Reed NL, Miller SJ, Gerstbrein J. Radioimmunoscintigraphy with In 111-labeled capromab pendetide predicts prostate cancer response to salvage radiotherapy after failed prostatectomy. *J Clin Oncol*. 1998;16:284–289.

9. Thomas CT, Bradshaw PT, Pollock BH, et al. Indium-111-capromab pendetide radioimmunoscintigraphy and prognosis for durable biochemical response to radiation therapy in men after failed prostatectomy. *J Clin Oncol*. 2003;21: 1715–1721.

10. Bott SRJ. Management of recurrent disease after radical prostatectomy. *Prostate Cancer Prostatic Dis*. 2004;7:211–216.

11. Pound CR, Partin AW, Epstein JI, Walsh PC. Prostate-specific antigen after anatomic radical retropubic prostatectomy. Patterns of recurrence and cancer control. *Urol Clin North Am*. 1997;24:395–406.

12. Roberts SG, Blute ML, Bergstralh EJ, Slezak JM, Zincke H. Biochemical doubling time as a predictor of clinical progression after biochemical failure following radical prostatectomy for prostate cancer. *Mayo Clin Proc.* 2001;76:576–581.

13. Stephenson AJ, Shariat SF, Zelefsky MJ, et al. Salvage radiotherapy for recurrent prostate cancer after radical prostatectomy. *JAMA.* 2004;291:1325–1332.

14. Stephenson AJ, Scardino PT, Kattan MW, et al. Predicting the outcome of salvage radiation therapy for recurrent prostate cancer after radical prostatectomy. *J Clin Oncol.* 2007;(25)15:2035–41.

15. Cox JD, Gallagher MJ, Hammond EH, Kaplan RS, Schell-hammer PF. Consensus statements on radiation therapy of prostate cancer: guidelines for prostate re-biopsy after radiation and for radiation therapy with rising prostate-specific antigen levels after radical prostatectomy. American Society for Therapeutic Radiology and Oncology Consensus Panel. *J Clin Oncol.* 1999;17:1155.

16. Trock BJ, Han M, Freedland SJ, Humphreys EB, DeWeese TL, Partin AW, Walsh PC. Prostate cancer-specific survival following salvage radiotherapy vs observation in men with biochemical recurrence after radical prostatectomy. *JAMA.* 2008 Jun 18;299(23):2760–9.

17. Ward JF, Sebo TJ, Blute ML, Zincke H. Salvage surgery for radiocurrent prostate cancer: contemporary outcomes. *J Urol.* 2005;173:1156–1160.

18. Stephenson AJ, Eastham JA. Role of salvage radical prostatectomy for recurrent prostate cancer after radiation therapy. *J Clin Oncol.* 2005;23:8198–8203.

19. Beyer DC. Salvage brachytherapy after external-beam irradiation for prostate cancer. *Oncology* (Williston Park). 2004;18:151–158.

20. Bahn DK, Lee F, Silverman P, et al. Salvage cryosurgery for recurrent prostate cancer after radiation therapy: a seven-year follow-up. *Clin Prostate Cancer.* 2003;2:111–114.

Section V

Clinical States: Castrate and Noncastrate Metastatic Disease

CHAPTER 8

Hormone Therapy of Prostate Cancer

■ Introduction

Androgen-suppressive therapy (AST) or androgen-depriva-tion therapy (ADT) has been the mainstay of the manage-ment of advanced prostate cancer since 1941, when Huggins and Hodges first reported clinical improvement in patients undergoing castration.[1] Over the ensuing 60 years, surgi-cal castration, estrogens, antiandrogens, antiadrenal agents, GnRH analogs, and more recently, GnRH antagonists, have been added to the armamentarium used by clinicians to treat metastatic and advanced local prostate cancer (**Figure 8-1**). Targeting the androgen receptor, even in patients who have failed AST, has become feasible with the approval of the testosterone synthesis inhibitor abiraterone acetate and the development of several other novel agents in clinical trials, leading the oncology community to reconsider the concept of hormone resistance. This chapter reviews the principles of AST in the management of prostatic adenocarcinoma, and its practical use.

Patients who develop metastatic disease with noncastrate testosterone levels are considered to be in the noncastrate-metastatic state. They remain in that state, even after AST has been started, and stay in it until they show progression of disease and transition to the castrate-resistant metastatic state (or die of prostate cancer or non-cancer-related causes).

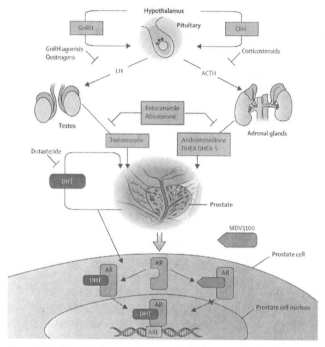

Figure 8-1 GnRH Analogs and Antagonist in Common Use in the U.S. Reprinted from *Lancet Oncology*, Vol. 10, Chen Y, et al. Anti-androgens and androgen-depleting therapies in prostate cancer: new agents for an established target, pages 981–991, copyright 2009, with permission from Elsevier.

■ Background

- ▪ Hypothalamic-pituitary-adrenal/gonadal axis
  - • LHRH (or GnRH), secreted by the hypothalamus in a pulsatile manner, stimulates the anterior pituitary gland to release luteinizing hormone (LH), which in turn stimulates the Leydig cells of the testes to produce testosterone.
  - • Within prostate epithelial cells, testosterone is converted by 5-alpha-reductase to the more potent ligand dihydrotestosterone (DHT), which has a four- to five-fold increased affinity for the androgen receptor (AR) compared with testosterone.

- DHT binds to the androgen receptor in the nucleus, which in turn binds to androgen-responsive genes, inducing transcription, promoting cellular growth, and inhibiting apoptosis.[2]
- The hypothalamic-pituitary-adrenal axis is another source of androgenic hormones. In response to cortico-tropin-releasing factor produced by the hypothalamus, the pituitary secretes adrenocorticotropic hormone (ACTH), which stimulates the adrenal gland to secrete dihydroepiandrosterone (DHEA), DHEA sulfate, and androstenedione. Although these are relatively weak androgens, their concentration in the blood is sufficiently high that after conversion to DHT within the prostate, they can amount to 40% of that hormone, the remaining 60% coming from testosterone secreted by the testes.[3]
- AST results in subjective and objective improvement in at least 80% of patients, with a median duration of response of 15–18 months.
- Eventually, androgen independence develops. Thus, hormone therapy is not curative. That these patients are not yet hormone refractory is evidenced by response to second- and third-line hormonal manipulations.
- Median survival from the time of first treatment of symptomatic disease is 2.5 years.[4] However, a great deal of variability in duration of response and survival after institution of AST can be seen, and some patients with advanced disease treated with hormones may survive 5–10 years.[5]
- The toxicity of hormonal therapy and its management is discussed later in greater detail.

■ Methods of Androgen Suppression

Bilateral Surgical Orchiectomy

- Method of action
  - Surgical extirpation of major site of testosterone production
- Technique
  - Subcapsular orchiectomy spares some scrotal contents but may leave residual testosterone-producing cells. Total orchiectomy is preferable.

- Advantages
  - Lower cost
  - Rapid induction of castrate state—testosterone levels decrease by 95% in 3 hours
  - Convenience—no need for further injections
- Disadvantages
  - Psychologically unacceptable to most men
  - Castration is permanent, leaving no option for intermittent therapy (see Continuous versus Intermittent Hormone Therapy, pp. 181)
  - Questionable impact on overall survival[6]

Estrogens

- Diethylstilbestrol (DES)
- Method of action
  - Estrogens suppress GnRH secretion from the hypothalamus through a negative feedback mechanism. LH levels fall, resulting in a decrease in serum testosterone to castrate levels in 2–9 weeks.[2,4]
- Advantages
  - Simple oral administration
  - Low cost
  - Testosterone levels suppressed without osteoporosis
  - No tumor flare
- Toxicity
  - Nausea, fluid retention, and feminization
  - Gynecomastia—may be prevented by radiation to the breasts
  - Increased mortality due to thromboembolic phenomena
    - The results of trials using prophylactic low-dose warfarin to prevent thromboembolic events have yielded conflicting results.[7]
- Efficacy
  - The results of several Veterans Administration Cooperative Urologic Research Group (VACURG) studies led to the following conclusions
    - Estrogens and orchiectomy are therapeutically equivalent.
    - DES 5 mg/day reduces cancer-specific mortality but increases mortality due to cardiovascular events.[6]

- DES 1 mg/day is equivalent in activity to DES 5 mg/day with no increase in cardiovascular toxicity in some, but not all, studies.[8] Other studies raise questions about the ability of lower doses of estrogens to adequately suppress testosterone.[9]
- Parenteral estrogens that avoid first-pass effect on clotting factor synthesis in the liver have been used but are not presently available in the United States.
- Estrogens: conclusion
  - Concern about thromboembolic events and availability of other agents has limited the use of estrogens in prostate cancer in the United States.
  - There is, however, renewed interest in the use of estrogens in the androgen-independent state.[10]

Tamoxifen and Selective Estrogen Receptor Modulators (SERMs)

- Tamoxifen
  - An estrogen receptor blocker shown to have modest activity in the early 1980s,[11] although endpoints were not clear. This agent is not commonly used.
- Raloxifene
  - A SERM currently under investigation

GnRH Agonists

- Mechanism of action
  - GnRH (also known as LHRH) agonists are synthetic compounds that mimic the endocrine signal from the hypothalamus to the pituitary gland that stimulate the production of gonadotropins.
  - After an initial increase in secretion of gonadotropins, pituitary receptors are down-regulated, decreasing gonadotropin secretion and resulting in castrate levels of circulating testosterone within 3–4 weeks.
  - The down-regulation of pituitary receptors is a result of continuous stimulation by the GnRH agonist, in contrast to the pulsatile stimulation that occurs naturally.

- Advantages
  - Safe and effective way to achieve castrate state
  - Psychologically more acceptable to most men than orchiectomy
  - No difference in response rate, time to progression, or survival compared with orchiectomy or DES in a variety of trials[3,12]
  - Reduction in testosterone levels in 2–3 weeks
  - Allows for the possibility of intermittent androgen suppression
  - Can be administered at intervals of as long as 4–12 months
- Disadvantages
  - Some preparations are painful when injected.
  - Initial increase in circulating testosterone can result in more rapid tumor growth, precipitating spinal cord compression, urinary tract obstruction, or severe pain flare.
    - 10–14 days of pretreatment with a peripheral anti-androgen, such as bicalutamide, flutamide, or nilutamide, can prevent tumor flare.
    - Newly available GnRH antagonists (degarelix) do not cause tumor flare and may reduce testosterone levels more rapidly.
- GnRH agonists conclusion
  - GnRH agonists are the most commonly used agents for hormone therapy. There is no evidence that any one agent is superior to the others (**Table 8-1**).

GnRH Antagonists

- Degarelix: a linear decapeptide that occupies GnRH receptor sites in the anterior pituitary gland
- Administration and dose: degarelix 240 mg (2 separate subcutaneous injections of 120 mg each) on day 1, followed by 80 mg subcutaneously every 28 days.
- Advantages
  - No testosterone flare that is seen with GnRH analogues
  - More rapid reduction of testosterone levels
  - No evidence of acute hypersensitivity reactions that were seen with abarelix, an earlier GnRH antagonist

Table 8-1 GnRH Agonists and Antagonist in Common Use in the U.S.

Name	Dose (mg)	Route	Frequency
GnRH Agonists			
Leuprolide acetate (Lupron Depot)	7.5	IM	Once monthly
	22.5	IM	q 3 months
	30.0	IM	q 4 months
Triptorelin pamoate (Trelstar®, Decapepty®)	3.75	IM	q month
	11.25	IM	q 3 months
Leuprolide acetate implant (Viadur®)	65.0	SQ	q 12 months*
Leuprolide acetate in Atrigel® Delivery System (Eligard®)	7.5	SQ	q month
	22.5	SQ	q 3 months
Goserelin acetate (Zoladex®)	3.6	SQ (abdominal wall)	q month
	10.8	SQ (abdominal wall)	q 3 months
GnRH Antagonist			
Degarelix (Firmagon®)	240 mg (two separate 120-mg injections) once only on day 1, then 80 mg	SQ	q month

*Requires surgical implantation

GnRH = gonadotropin-releasing hormone; IM = intramuscular; SQ = subcutaneous.

- Disadvantages
  - Monthly injections are required
  - Increased risk of local injection site reactions
  - Cost?
- Degarelix: supporting data
  - CS 21[13]
    - Randomized open-label, multi-institutional trial
    - 610 patients with all stages of prostate cancer
    - Arms
      - Degarelix 240 mg once followed by 80 mg monthly
      - Degarelix 240 mg once followed by 160 mg monthly
      - Leuprolide 7.5 mg monthly
    - Treatment continued for 12 months
    - It should be noted that this was a noninferiority trial
  - Primary endpoint
    - Cumulative probability of testosterone level less than or equal to 0.5 ng/mL at any monthly measurement from 28–364 days
  - Multiple secondary endpoints focusing on
    - Testosterone levels at various time points
    - PSA changes
    - Time to PSA progression
    - Adverse events and quality of life measures
  - Results
    - No difference in primary endpoint: percentage of patients achieving testosterone levels of ≤ 0.5 ng/mL
      - Degarelix 240/80 mg: 97%
      - Degarelix 240/160 mg: 98.3%
      - Leuprolide 7.5: 96.4%
    - No evidence of testosterone flare with degarelix
    - More rapid reduction in testosterone levels
      - At 3 days, 96% of patients receiving degarelix and none of the patients receiving leuprolide achieved testosterone levels of ≤ 0.5 ng/mL
      - After 28 days, testosterone levels were similar across groups
    - More rapid decline in PSA at 14 and 28 days for both degarelix groups compared with leuprolide (84% decrease in PSA for degarelix vs 68% for leuprolide)

- ▪ Degarelix was associated with more local skin reactions compared to leuprolide (40% vs. < 1%)
- ▪ No systemic allergic reactions seen
- ▪ Mild transaminitis seen in < 10% of all groups
- ▪ Other side effects were similar across groups
- • Conclusion
  - ▪ Degarelix is not inferior to leuprolide in maintaining testosterone suppression over a 1-year period.
- • Comment
  - ▪ Design of study did not allow evaluation of clinical benefit or tumor response other than by PSA.
- • Additional analysis of the data from CS 21 looking at PSA outcomes was published online.[57]
  - ▪ http://www.asco.org/ascov2/Meetings/Abstracts? &vmview=abst_detail_view&confID=64 &abstractID=20342
  - ▪ The overall risk of PSA failure (during 1 year) was less for degarelix 240/80 (7.7%) compared to degarelix 240/160 (12.9%) and leuprolide (12.9%)
    - • It is unclear why degarelix 240/160 appears inferior to degarelix 240/80 or leuprolide.
  - ▪ Degarelix reduced PSA more rapidly than leuprolide.
    - • At 28 days, 59% of patients getting degarelix had PSA levels < 4.0 ng/ml compared to 34% for patients getting leuprolide.
    - • By day 364 the difference (83% vs. 78%) was not significant; p = 0.339.
  - ▪ Patients receiving degarelix had a statistically significant decrease (2%) in the risk of death during the year on study compared with those receiving leuprolide (4%); p = 0.05.
- • An extension study was reported as an abstract at the 2011 ASCO Genitourinary Cancers Symposium and recently published[44]
  - ▪ Patients originally randomized to leuprolide were offered randomization to continued leuprolide vs degarelix 240 mg for 1 month followed by either 80 or 160 mg per month.

- At 1 year the risk of PSA progression and death was significantly lower for patients switched to degarelix 240/80 compared to those who remained on leuprolide.
- *Comment*:
  - Degarelix, a pure GnRH antagonist should be considered as initial therapy for those patients in whom a rapid induction of the castrate state, without risk of testosterone flare, is needed.
  - These are usually hormone-naïve or noncastrate patients who present with emergent symptoms such as pain crisis, impending or actual spinal cord compression, urinary or bowel obstruction or coagulopathies (DIC alone or with excessive fibrinolysis).
  - Other options to consider in that situation might include high-dose ketoconazole or surgical castration.
  - It is not known whether or not patients failing a GnRH analog would benefit from a change to degarelix
  - Whether or not degarelix is superior to GnRH agonists in the long term is not yet known.

Antiandrogens

- Antiandrogens are useful because surgical castration and GnRH agonists or antagonists do not completely eliminate androgens, particularly those originating in the adrenal gland.
  - Steroidal antiandrogens—cyproterone acetate, megestrol acetate, and medroxyprogesterone acetate, mifeprestone, spironolactone
    - Mechanism of action
      - Inhibition of gonadotropin release
      - Androgen receptor blockade (ARB)
      - Reduced synthesis of adrenal androgens
      - Advantages
      - Inexpensive
      - Progestational activity prevents hot flashes
      - Less thrombogenic than estrogens
    - Disadvantages
      - Cyproterone is not approved for prostate cancer in the United States.
      - Weight gain, fluid retention, and hepatotoxicity

- Megestrol acetate may be less effective and may increase risk of thromboembolic events.
- Some clinicians avoid the use of progestational agents and spironolactone because of concern that they can stimulate growth of prostate cancer cells.
- Steroidal antiandrogens conclusion
  - Steroidal antiandrogens are not commonly used in the United States.
- Nonsteroidal antiandrogens
  - Mechanism of action
    - High affinity for androgen receptor results in effective blockade by inducing conformational changes that inhibit transcription.
    - Blocking of effect of androgen on the hypothalamus and pituitary causes increased secretion of LH and consequent increase in testosterone secretion.
  - Advantages
    - Simple oral administration
    - Effect on overall survival similar to orchiectomy[12]
    - Avoids some symptoms caused by AST
      - Libido and potency preserved when used as single agents
    - Useful prior to administration of GnRH agonists in order to prevent flare
  - Disadvantages
    - Lower affinity of nonsteroidal antiandrogens for androgen receptor compared with testosterone and DHT may allow drug to be displaced, resulting in suboptimal androgen blockade when used as single agents.
    - Hepatotoxicity, breast enlargement and tenderness, diarrhea
  - Flutamide
    - Dose: 250 mg PO three times daily
    - Toxicity
      - Diarrhea (26%)
      - Gynecomastia
      - Hepatotoxicity

- Nilutamide
  - Dose: 150 mg twice daily for first month, 150 mg once daily thereafter
  - Toxicity
    - Alcohol intolerance (antabuse effect)
    - Visual—difficulty with light–dark adjustment
    - Rare lung toxicity
- Bicalutamide
  - Dose
    - 50 mg once daily
    - 150 mg once daily has shown equivalence to castration for patients with localized disease, but this dose level is not approved by the U.S. Food and Drug Administration (FDA).[14]
      - High-dose bicalutamide (150 mg/day) has also been studied in the adjuvant setting and found to delay progression after radical prostatectomy and radiotherapy.[15] However, an increase in deaths among patients receiving high-dose bicalutamide compared with those receiving placebo in another trial raised sufficient concern that bicalutamide at 150 mg/day is no longer approved in Great Britain and Canada.[16]
  - Toxicity[17]
    - Gynecomastia and breast tenderness due to conversion of excess testosterone to estrogens and increased prolactin levels
      - Prophylactic low-dose (10 Gy) radiotherapy to the breasts may lower the risk of gynecomastia and breast pain.
      - Gynecomastia may or may not resolve upon cessation of bicalutamide, depending on duration of therapy.
      - Established gynecomastia can be treated with reductive surgery.
      - The role of antiestrogens in the treatment and prevention of these symptoms is under investigation.

- Increased sensitivity to warfarin, because bicalutamide displaces warfarin from binding proteins
- Diarrhea (12%) less likely compared with flutamide
- Alcohol intolerance and visual disturbances not reported
- Rare elevations of liver function studies usually normalize with cessation of therapy.
- Antiandrogen withdrawal response
  - Approximately 25–30% of patients experiencing disease progression on nonsteroidal antiandrogen therapy respond to withdrawal of those agents.[18]
  - In addition to PSA level declines, decrease in measurable disease and improvement in symptoms may be seen.
    - Although these responses may be brief, in some patients they are sufficient to allow a delay in institution of chemotherapy for several months.
    - The mechanism of this response probably relates to mutations in the androgen receptor that cause the antiandrogen to act as a growth promoter rather than a growth inhibitor.
  - Secondary and tertiary hormone therapy
    - Clinicians caring for patients who experience treatment failure with GnRH agonist or antagonist and a nonsteroidal antiandrogen often consider further attempts at hormonal manipulation in order to avoid the toxicity of chemotherapy, particularly in patients who are asymptomatic, have biochemical failure alone, or have small-volume metastases.
    - For these patients it is reasonable to try a different antiandrogen once the patient progresses through, or fails to respond to, withdrawal of the original antiandrogen.
    - Response rates between 14% and 50% have been reported with niluatmide[19] and higher doses of bicalutamide.[20] A response to antiandrogen withdrawal increases the likelihood of response to second-line antiandrogens.

- New antiandrogens: MDV 3100
  - Novel androgen receptor antagonist given orally
    - Blocks androgens from binding to the androgen receptor (AR)
    - Higher affinity for the AR than bicalutamide
    - Impairs nuclear transcription, DNA binding, and coactivator recruitment
    - Induces apoptosis
    - Lacks agonist activity
  - Phase 1–2 study[45]
    - Patient characteristics
      - 140 patients with castrate-resistant prostate cancer in a multicenter dose escalation (30–600 mg per day) study
      - 54% had prior chemotherapy.
      - Most patients with detectable disease had bone or lymph node involvement; only 9% had visceral involvement.
      - 5% had biochemical failure only.
    - Results
      - Overall, 55% of patients had a 50% or greater drop in PSA.
        - Response rates were similar for prior chemo and no prior chemo groups.
        - Chemotherapy-naïve patients responded more quickly.
      - 25 of 51 (49%) had drop in circulating tumor cell counts from levels considered unfavorable to levels considered favorable.
      - 13 of 59 (22%) had response in soft tissue.
      - 61 of 109 patients (56%) had stable bone disease.
      - Decreased binding of DHT to AR was demonstrated by fDHT PET scanning in all of the 22 patients studied.
      - MTD was 240 mg/day.
      - Median time to PSA progression was 27 weeks for patients who had received prior chemotherapy but was not reached for the entire cohort.

- Median time to radiological progression was 47 weeks; 95% CI (20–not reached).
- Grade 3 or 4 fatigue was seen in approximately 20% of patients receiving daily doses of 240–280 mg.
  - Fatigue usually resolved within 2–4 weeks of dose reduction.
- Three patients had seizures that were thought to be unrelated to therapy.
- Conclusion, MDV 3100
  - MDV 3100 is an active and well tolerated anti-androgen in men with castrate-resistant prostate cancer.
  - Randomized placebo-controlled Phase 3 trials are either underway or recently completed in both the chemotherapy-naïve and post-docetaxel populations.
- ARN 509
  - An oral antiandrogen currently under investigation[46]
  - Analog of MDV
  - Targets overexpressed androgen receptor
  - More potent and more effective anti androgen in pre-clinical trials[47]
- Antiandrogens conclusion
  - The availability of nonsteroidal antiandrogens has limited the use of steroidal agents in the United States. Ease of use and avoidance of symptoms related to testosterone deprivation are attractive to patients with prostate cancer and their physicians, but cost and suboptimal androgen blockade when used alone limit their use as single agents.
  - These drugs are generally used prior to institution of a GnRH agonist to prevent tumor flare, or in conjunction with GnRH agonists as part of a combined or maximal androgen blockade.
  - The use of these drugs as single agents, in the adjuvant setting or in combination with finasteride, remains investigational and is discussed elsewhere.

Inhibitors of Testosterone Synthesis

- These agents prevent the synthesis of steroids that can be converted to testosterone, and eventually DHT, in the prostate gland.
- Ketoconazole
  - An imidazole antifungal agent with reported response rates (50% decrease in PSA levels) as high as 62% in patients who fail antiandrogen withdrawal.[21]
  - Mechanism of action
    - Inhibits gonadal and adrenal androgen synthesis
  - Dose
    - 400 mg three times per day
    - Some clinicians begin at lower doses (200 mg three times per day) and gradually escalate to full doses as tolerated.
    - Should not be taken with food, antacids, proton pump inhibitors, or histamine-2 receptor blockers to maximize absorption and bioavailability
    - Replacement doses of hydrocortisone (20–40 mg/day) should be given.
  - Advantages
    - Rapid achievement of castrate state makes this agent useful in emergent situations, particularly if the patient is hormone naïve.
    - Simple oral administration
  - Disadvantages/toxicity[4]
    - Adrenal insufficiency
    - Nausea and vomiting
    - Hepatotoxicity (10%)
    - Short half-life and q 8-hour dosing require strict compliance in order to avoid a breakthrough increase in steroid synthesis.
    - Inhibition of the P450 cytochrome pathway requires attention to the possibility of interaction with other drugs the patient may be taking.
- Finasteride and dutasteride
  - Competitive inhibitors of 5-alpha reductase commonly used for the treatment of obstructive symptoms due to BPH and, in lower doses, for the treatment of male pattern baldness.

- Prevents conversion of testosterone to DHT, a stronger ligand of the androgen receptor
- These agents have been investigated as preventative agents (see Chapter 1) and in combination with bicalutamide for biochemical failure after surgery or radiotherapy.
- Some data suggest that 5-alpha reductase inhibitors may slow progression of prostate cancer in men on active surveillance.
- The role for these agents in the treatment of advanced prostate cancer remains undefined.
- New testosterone synthesis inhibitors: abiraterone acetate
  - Abiraterone acetate (AA) is a new selective androgen synthesis inhibitor that blocks CYP 17 A, decreasing the production of androgens from the adrenal gland and intratumoral sources.
  - Cougar-AA-301 is a randomized, double-blind, controlled trial comparing AA 1000 mg/day plus prednisone 5 mg twice daily to placebo plus the same dose of prednisone.[48]
    - 1195 patients who have received no more than two chemotherapy regimens one of which must be docetaxel.
    - Prior ketoconazole was not allowed.
    - Primary endpoint is overall survival (OS).
  - Results
    - OS was significantly better for AA + prednisone versus Placebo + prednisone such that the trial was unblinded and stopped after a planned interim analysis that revealed:
      - OS for patients receiving abiraterone plus prednisone was 14.8 months
      - OS for patient receiving placebo plus prednisone was 10.9 months
      - HR 0.646, 95% CI (0.54–0.77), $p \leq 0.0001$

- Adverse events largely due to increase in mineralocorticoid and other steroids upstream from the CYP17A blockade
  * Edema: 31%
  * Hypokalemia: 17%
  * Hypertension: 10%
  * Cardiac: 13%
  * Hepatic: 10%
- The dose is 1000 mg (four 250 mg tabs) taken at the same time once daily.
- The dose should be reduced for severe hepatic dysfunction.
- Conclusions:
  - Abiraterone acetate plus prednisone is a well tolerated active treatment for men with castrate-resistant prostate cancer who have progressed through at least one docetaxel-based chemotherapy regimen and no more than two prior chemotherapy regimens.
  - A similar Phase 3 trial was just completed for patients who are chemotherapy naïve; it is no longer accruing patients.
  - In the spring of 2011, abiraterone acetate was approved by the FDA for treatment of castrate-resistant prostate cancer in patients who have received docetaxel.
  - The results of studies using abiraterone acetate in patients who have not received docetaxel are eagerly awaited.
- TAK-700—Currently investigational[49]
  - Selective inhibitor of 17–20 lyase which results in decreased production of androgenic steroids
  - 96 patients with castration-reistant prostate cancer and no prior chemotherapy.
  - 41–63% of patients (depending on dose level) had 50% reduction in PSA
  - Median testosterone and dehydroepiandrosterone levels dropped at all dose levels at 12 weeks
  - 6/43 evaluable patients had partial response by RECIST criteria

- Toxicity (less than 10% grade 3) included
  - Fatigue
  - Nausea
  - Constipation
  - 13% withdrew from trial because of side affects

Other Hormonal Agents

- Corticosteroids
  - Corticosteroids are widely used for patients with advanced prostate cancer.
    - High doses of dexamethasone are commonly used in the management of spinal cord compression or other neurologic emergencies.
    - Low doses of prednisone (10–20 mg/day) may effectively reduce pain, increase appetite, and improve the patient's overall sense of well-being.[22]
- Progestational agents
  - Megestrol acetate has minor activity in hormone-refractory disease.[23] Concern about thromboembolic events and the possibility of promotion of tumor growth limits its use.

■ Controversies in Hormone Therapy

Combined Androgen Blockade (CAB) Versus Monotherapy

- Surgical or medical castration may reduce the amount of 5-alpha-DHT available to the prostate cancer cell by only 60%.
- The response rate seen with that inhibit androgen synthesis in patients experiencing treatment failure with primary hormone therapy suggests that DHT derived from adrenal steroids and from the small amount of testosterone produced in the prostate may be enough to stimulate the growth of prostate cancer cells. Overexpression of AR and other adaptations create further opportunities for therapeutic intervention with novel agents. The experience with MDV 3100 and abiraterone acetate support this concept
  - The addition of flutamide to leuprolide was shown to delay progression by 2.6 months and improve overall survival by 7.3 months compared with leuprolide alone.[24]

- No advantage was found in a SWOG study for the addition of flutamide to orchiectomy.[25] Other trials, particularly those in which surgical castration was used, yielded conflicting results.
  - A large meta-analysis revealed a very modest (less than 3%), but significant, improvement in 5-year survival for those getting flutamide or nilutamide in addition to surgical or medical castration. No significant advantage, in fact, inferior survival was seen with cyproterone.[26]
- Based on the results of a large meta-analysis, bicalutamide, another nonandrogen which is better tolerated, may offer a 20% (95% CI of 0.66–0.98) survival advantage when used in combination with a GnRH agonist compared to a GnRH agonist alone.[50]
- CAB versus monotherapy: conclusion.
  - The addition of certain peripheral nonsteroidal antiandrogens to medical or surgical castration offers a minor survival advantage.
  - If combined androgen blockade is used, the preferred antiandrogen is bicalutamide. This is based on data from a meta-analysis.
  - Bicalutamide is generally well tolerated compared to other antiandrogens.
  - With the availability of generic bicalutamide and the expected reduction in cost of the drug, one of the major impediments to CAB is eliminated.
  - Some clinicians recommend combined androgen blockade as standard initial therapy, but the issue remains controversial and is unlikely to be resolved by prospective trials. Guidelines from professional organizations vary. The National Comprehensive Cancer Network (NCCN) recommends monotherapy without an antiandrogen as initial therapy.
  - For an in depth discussion of this issue please see Chodak 2007.[51]

Early Versus Delayed Hormone Therapy

■ Because of the inevitable emergence of androgen independence, hormone therapy is palliative rather than curative. Thus, benefits of this treatment have to be carefully weighed against expected toxicity, particularly in patients who are either asymptomatic or minimally symptomatic from their disease.

■ Because many of the patients considered for hormone therapy have either biochemical (PSA) failure alone, or manifest but small-volume asymptomatic metastases detected by PSA level, this becomes an important quality-of-life issue.

■ The use of hormone therapy in patients with rising PSA levels after primary therapy or biochemical failure and in the adjuvant or neoadjuvant setting is discussed elsewhere. The principle of early institution of hormone therapy is based on several trials:

  • VACURG studies comparing orchiectomy, various doses of DES, and observation suggested that young patients with high-grade disease or stage T3 tumors benefit from early institution of hormone therapy.

    ■ These studies were confounded to some extent by the increased cardiovascular mortality seen with higher doses of DES.[27]

  • Medical Research Council studies looked at immediate versus delayed hormone therapy (orchiectomy or GnRH agonist) in patients with advanced local or asymptomatic metastatic disease.

    ■ Progression to metastatic disease (among those with advanced local tumors) and development of pain in patients who were initially asymptomatic occurred later in immediately treated patients compared with those in whom treatment was started when symptoms occurred.

    ■ A survival benefit was also seen for early institution of hormone therapy.

      • These studies were criticized because some patients never received hormone therapy or were treated only after significant complications of their disease developed. Thus, interpretation of the survival data is difficult.[28]

- EORTC reported a survival advantage for patients with locally advanced prostate cancer given a GnRH analog at the commencement of radiotherapy and continuing for 3 years compared with those treated with radiotherapy alone.[29]
- RTOG examined the benefit of adjuvant goserelin after radiotherapy for locally advanced prostate cancer and found improved local control and freedom from progression over radiotherapy alone.
  - A significant survival advantage was seen only for patients with high-grade tumors (Gleason scores of 8–10).[30]
- ECOG randomized patients found to have positive nodes at the time of radical prostatectomy to either immediate hormone therapy or observation. Significant improvement in survival was seen for the immediately treated group.[31]
- A retrospective study looked at early vs. delayed institution of androgen suppressive therapy in patients with PSA failure after prostatectomy.[52]
  - Overall, there was no difference in time to clinical metastases
  - However, in the subset of patients with Gleason scores of 7 or higher and a doubling time of 12 months or less, time to clinical metastases was improved in the early androgen suppression group.
- Early versus delayed hormone therapy conclusions
  - Trials are difficult to interpret because many were adjuvant studies, or studies done on patients with advanced local disease. Most were retrospective.
  - There is no consensus on the optimal timing of the institution of androgen suppressive therapy for patients with pure biochemical failure (absence of detectable recurrence or metastases).

- There may be a benefit for early institution of hormone therapy, particularly in patients with high-grade disease and a rapid doubling time.
  - However, significant changes in quality of life accompany hormone therapy, and the benefits may be modest. Patients who are subjected to androgen suppressive therapy for PSA failure alone of for small volume asymptomatic metastases should be considered for intermittent rather than continuous therapy.
  - This represents another example of a treatment decision that must be carefully discussed with the patient. Some men may insist on institution of therapy at the very first sign of progression. Others may choose to defer treatment in order to preserve sexual function and avoid other toxicities.
- Clearly, the development of better predictive tools is needed to help men and their physicians facing this decision.
- NCCN guidelines currently advise that patients with PSA levels > 50 ng/ml and those with PSA–doubling times less than 12 months should be offered androgen-suppressive therapy because they face a higher risk of death from prostate cancer.[58] But the data in support of that recommendation come from a study in patients without metastatic disease who were not candidates for curative therapy.

Continuous Versus Intermittent Hormone Therapy[53]

- With the advent of medical castration, the possibility of intermittent testosterone suppression became feasible.
  - Animal studies suggest that intermittent androgen blockade may delay the onset of hormone-resistant disease.[32]
  - A small Belgian trial[33] that enrolled primarily patients with advanced local disease showed a significantly lower progression rate for intermittent versus continuous therapy.

- A variety of trials that included a heterogeneous patient population undergoing AST in different ways provides tentative evidence for the feasibility of intermittent therapy.
  - Most of the trials are single institutional small studies.
  - These trials have observed continuing efficacy of AST when reinstituted after significant time off treatment.[34]
- While larger randomized clinical trials are underway, none have been completed and thus no firm guidelines exist.
- For patients expressing interest in intermittent therapy, the lack of data supporting the intermittent approach should be emphasized. At the time of initial institution of hormone therapy, it should be emphasized to patients that discontinuation of therapy may not result in a rebound in testosterone levels and consequent improvement in symptoms related to testosterone deprivation.
  - With those caveats, it would be reasonable to stop androgen suppressive therapy after 8–10 months, assuming that the PSA level has plateaued and the patient feels well.
- The indications for restarting hormone therapy are also unsettled.
  - A PSA trigger point of 10 ng/ml is commonly used in clinical trials, but that number is arbitrary.
  - Other studies have used a PSA level that is 50% of the level present when hormone therapy was stopped.
  - As is true in many areas of prostate cancer treatment, the timing of the resumption of hormone therapy may be more a function of patient or physician anxiety than of science.
  - The uncertainties surrounding intermittent androgen therapy were nicely reviewed in a paper by Shore and Crawford in 2010.[54]
  - Two trials that are currently underway—SWOG9346 (NCIC PR8) and SWOG/NCIC JPR7—may help resolve this question.

- Duration of androgen-suppressive therapy
  - It is common practice to maintain patients on androgen suppression indefinitely, either on a continuous or intermittent basis.
  - The rationale behind this approach is based on the assumption that some androgen-dependent clones remain despite the emergence of androgen-independent cells.
  - It would not be unreasonable to stop medical castration in patients with end-stage disease in order to spare them the cost, discomfort, and inconvenience attendant to GnRH agonist or antagonist therapy.

■ Complications of AST

- Hot flashes
  - Hot flashes develop in almost all patients undergoing AST for prostate cancer.[35]
  - They can occur at night or during the day and may be associated with significant sweating.
  - For the vast majority of men, they are a minor nuisance. However, in somewhere between 5% and 10% of men undergoing androgen suppression, pharmacologic intervention or, in rare cases, discontinuation of therapy is needed.
  - Pharmacologic intervention
    - Estrogens
      - DES is no longer available.
      - Estradiol transdermal system of patches delivering 0.025 mg/d, applied q 7 days, has been used by some clinicians.
    - Progestins
      - Megestrol acetate
        - Dose: 20–40 mg/day
        - Highly effective in relieving hot flashes,[36] but there is concern that this agent may cause progression of disease, edema, and thromboembolic events
      - Steroidal antiandrogens: cyproterone acetate 100 mg daily

- Miscellaneous
  - Clonidine
    - Starting dose of 0.1 mg/day
    - Evidence for efficacy is anecdotal. Placebo-controlled trials have been negative in outcome.
  - Venlafaxine (a selective serotonin reuptake inhibitor)
    - Dose: 37.5–75 mg/day
    - Treatment of cancer-associated depression is an additional benefit.
    - In one randomized trial, venlafaxine reduced hot flash symptoms by 47%. But results for cyproterone and megestrol acetate were better, 95% and 84% respectively.[55]
- Alternative and complementary therapy
  - Acupuncture
  - Soy
    - More bioavailable soy in soybeans than in soymilk and soy powder
  - Vitamin E
- Osteoporosis
  - Men undergoing AST are known to develop significant loss of bone mineral density and to show signs of increased bone turnover. This results in a two-and-one-half-fold increase in the risk of bone fracture compared with rates observed in the general population.[37]
  - General preventive measures
    - Possible intermittent androgen ablation
    - Exercise
    - Calcium supplementation (800–1,500 mg/day)
    - Vitamin D (800–1200 IU/day)
    - Monitoring with bone densitometry
      - Exact role not yet defined
  - Bisphosphonates
    - Mechanism of action is to decrease resorption of bone by osteoclast inhibition

* Available agents
  * Alendronate 70 mg PO once weekly
    * Must be taken on empty stomach
    * Patient must remain upright for 30 minutes after ingesting pill
  * Pamidronate 60 mg IV every 12 weeks
  * Zoledronate 4 mg IV in at least 100 cc of IV fluids over 15 minutes
    * Dose should be reduced in patients with renal insufficiency.
    * **Although there is evidence that bisphosphonates reduce bone loss in patients receiving AST, there are no randomized trials showing that they prevent skeletal complications in the nonmetastatic state. Thus, the indication for use of these agents and the optimal frequency of their administration in the nonmetastatic state remain undefined.**
    * Both pamidronate and zoledronate have been shown to prevent bone loss but they have not yet been proven to reduce or delay skeletal related events, in patients undergoing AST, for nonmetastatic prostate cancer.[38,39]
  * Toxicity
    * Low-grade fever
    * Arthralgia and myalgia
    * Cytopenias
    * Constipation
    * Hypocalcemia and hypophosphatemia
    * Decreased renal function
    * Higher doses and rapid infusion increase toxicity risk.
    * When zoledronate 4 mg is administered as described earlier, the risk of significant increase in creatinine is less than 2%.
      * Dose should be adjusted for renal function and renal function should be monitored.
    * Radiation recall effect
    * Osteonecrosis of the jaw (see Chapter 9)

- Denosumab
  - Denosumab is a new monoclonal antibody against the receptor activator of nuclear factor ß ligand.
  - At doses of 60 mg subcutaneously every 6 months given to men receiving androgen-suppressive therapy for nonmetastatic prostate cancer, bone mineral density was improved compared to placebo and the incidence of vertebral fractures was reduced. Adverse events were similar in both groups (denosumab vs. placebo).[56]
  - At the higher doses used for castrate-resistant prostate cancer (see Chapter 9), severe (grade 3 and 4) hypocalcemia and hypophosphatemia have been observed (personal communication with Michael Morris, MD). Guidelines for using this agent are evolving. Patients should be taking calcium and vitamin D replacement. The role of serum calcium, phosphorous, and vitamin D levels before and during treatment with denosumab is not yet defined. The drug should either not be used at all or used with great caution in patients with a glomerular filtration rate of less than 30 ml/min.
  - Conclusion: Denosumab 60 mg subcutaneously every 6 months may delay skeletal complications in men undergoing androgen suppressive therapy for non-metastatic, biochemical failure.
  - The use of these agents in patients with manifest bone metastases is discussed in Chapter 9.
- Fatigue and anemia
  - Mild normocytic, normochromic, anemia is commonly seen during AST.
  - Fatigue, as reported by patients, may be out of proportion to the degree of anemia.
  - **Other causes of anemia should be excluded.**
  - When fatigue does not improve with the correction of anemia, and no other cause has been identified, consideration should be given to the use of antidepressants or modafinil.

- Sexual dysfunction
  - Reduction in serum testosterone to castrate levels almost always results in erectile difficulties and (perhaps thankfully) decreased libido.
  - Many patients treated with hormone therapy already suffer from some degree of sexual dysfunction because of prior surgery and radiotherapy or because of complications of their cancer, such as advanced locoregional disease, pain, genital swelling, depression, and fatigue.
  - While exogenous testosterone is currently under investigation in advanced prostate cancer, it remains contraindicated for the treatment of sexual dysfunction or hot flashes due to androgen suppression.
  - Few clinical trials have addressed the problem of erectile dysfunction, but the following techniques have been used
    - Sildenafil, tadalafil, or vardenafil when no contraindications exist
    - Intracavernous injection of alprostadil
    - Vacuum pump can be effective but not always acceptable
    - Penile prosthesis
  - In those patients for whom sexual dysfunction is an unacceptable quality-of-life issue and who experience failure with the modalities discussed earlier, intermittent hormone therapy should be considered when feasible.
- Gynecomastia
  - Incidence is greater with CAB (50%) than with GnRH therapy alone (25%). The greatest risk is with antiandrogens alone.
  - Low-dose radiotherapy to the breasts can prevent gynecomastia or reduce its severity but is ineffective once breast enlargement develops.
    - The risk of a radiotherapy-induced breast cancer limits the usefulness of this approach in patients who are being treated in the adjuvant or neoadjuvant setting.

* In severe cases, reduction mammoplasty can be considered.
* The role of antiestrogens, such as tamoxifen, either given prophylactically or as therapy remains undefined.
▪ Other side effects of AST
  * Change in body habitus and weight gain
  * Atrophy of testicles and reduction in penile size
  * Loss of body hair
  * Cognitive defects
  * Muscle weakness
  * Insomnia
  * Depression, mood swings
  * Increased cholesterol or triglycerides

■ Summary and Practical Use of AST

▪ AST is an effective treatment for advanced symptomatic prostate cancer, with acceptable toxicity, for the vast majority of patients.

▪ Therapy may be deferred for some patients with biochemical failure only and those with asymptomatic, small-volume disease, because the impact of early treatment on survival is small.[40]

* The optimal timing of androgen-suppressive therapy remains controversial for patients in whom the only sign of disease is an increasing PSA level. Patient and doctor anxiety frequently lead to early institution of therapy with modest long-term benefit at the expense of significant quality of life changes. The advantages and disadvantages should be discussed with the patient and delay in treatment should be encouraged unless the patient has symptomatic recurrence or extensive disease by imaging.

* Patients with rapid doubling times, high grade disease, or absolute PSA values greater than 50 ng/mL should be made aware of the data predicting earlier rather than later symptomatic relapse and the advantages/disadvantages should be discussed.

- Before starting GnRH agonist therapy, patients at risk for tumor flare should receive 10–14 days of an antiandrogen, such as flutamide, bicalutamide, or nilutamide. Once the risk of flare has passed (usually within 2–4 weeks after the start of GnRH agonist therapy), the antiandrogen may be discontinued.

- Patients needing more urgent androgen suppression may be treated with degarelix, a GnRH antagonist, or with surgical castration. Alternatively, treatment with high-dose ketoconazole and replacement doses of hydrocortisone, as described earlier, can be started concurrent with the institution of an antiandrogen. In this case, ketoconazole and hydrocortisone should be continued until the GnRH agonist can be given and for a few weeks after.

- The use of combined androgen blockade versus GnRH agonist or antagonist therapy alone remains controversial. If a nonsteroidal antiandrogen is used in conjunction with medical castration, is should be bicalutamide.

- A peripheral nonsteroidal antiandrogen, preferably bicalutamide, should be added to the regimen for patients experiencing disease progression on GnRH agonist monotherapy.

- There is no evidence that switching from one GnRH agonist to another or from medical castration to surgical orchiectomy results in a secondary response.

- For patients with disease failing CAB, the antiandrogen should be discontinued and the patient should be monitored for an antiandrogen withdrawal response.

- Patients whose disease fails to respond to antiandrogen withdrawal who are asymptomatic can be observed or offered second-line hormone therapy with ketoconazole. On occasion, responses may be seen after changing to a different antiandrogen. The availability of newer agents such as abiraterone acetate and MDV 3100 may provide even more options in this setting

- For patients who fail second- or third-line hormonal manipulations, chemotherapy, palliative radiotherapy, or even systemic radioisotopes can be considered (see Chapter 9).

- Although intermittent androgen suppression remains experimental pending the outcome of randomized controlled trials, it should be considered for patient with biochemical failure alone or those with small volume asymptomatic metastases.

- At all decision-making points, careful assessment of the risk-benefit ratio of the proposed treatment should be made. Where therapy is palliative, toxicity should be avoided, particularly when the patient is asymptomatic or minimally symptomatic.

The Transition to the Castrate-Resistant State

- Although almost all patients with prostate cancer respond to AST to some degree, the emergence of androgen independence is inevitable.

- Thus, AST is not curative.

- Despite the development of the androgen-independent state, the androgen receptor (AR) signaling pathway is maintained.

- Mechanisms of androgen resistance[34,41–43]
  - Selection of preexisting resistant cells by AST
    - These cells may derive from basal-layer "stem cells" that are not intrinsically androgen dependent.
  - Activation of survival pathways
  - Amplification and overexpression of the AR, resulting in increased sensitivity of the AR to low levels of circulating androgens
  - Mutations causing altered ligand specificity, allowing activation by nonandrogens or antiandrogens
  - Insulin-like growth factor, keratinocyte growth factor, and epidermal growth factor may activate receptor tyrosine kinases, resulting in phosphorylation of AR by protein kinase B (Akt), or mitogen-activated protein kinase.
  - Increased antiapoptotic pathways (e.g., mediated by bcl-2)

- For these reasons, the terms androgen independent and hormone refractory may be misleading. The clinical status of patients who progress while on AST is better described as castrate resistant (see Chapter 1).

■ References

1. Huggins C, Hodges CV. Studies in prostatic cancer II. The effect of castration on advanced carcinoma of the prostate gland. *Arch Surg.* 1941;43:209–223.

2. Petrylak DP, Moul JW. Androgen ablation for prostate cancer: mechanisms and modalities. In: Kantoff PW, Carroll PR, D'Amico AV, eds. *Prostate Cancer: Principles and Practice.* Philadelphia: Lippincott Williams and Wilkins; 2002:518–523.

3. Schellhammer PF. Combined androgen blockade for the treatment of metastatic cancer of the prostate. In: Kantoff PW, Carroll PR, D' Amico AV, eds. *Prostate Cancer: Principles and Practice.* Philadelphia: Lippincott Williams and Wilkins; 2002:524–540.

4. Galbraith SM, Duchesne GM. Androgens and prostate cancer: biology, pathology and hormonal therapy. *Eur J Cancer.* 1997;33:545–554.

5. Crawford ED, Rosenblum M, Ziada AM, Lange PH. Hormone refractory prostate cancer. *Urology.* 1999;54(suppl):1–7.

6. Veterans Administration Co-operative Urological Research Group. Treatment and survival of patients with cancer of the prostate. *Surg Gynecol Obstet.* 1967;124:1011–1017.

7. Klotz L, McNeill I, Fleisher N. A phase 1/2 trial of diethylstilbestrol plus low dose warfarin in advanced prostate carcinoma. *J Urol.* 1999;161:169–172.

8. Cox RL, Crawford ED. Estrogens in the treatment of prostate cancer. *J Urol.* 1995;154:1991–1998.

9. Malkowicz S. The role of diethylstilbestrol in the treatment of prostate cancer. *Urology.* 2001;58(suppl 1):108–113.

10. Oh WK. The evolving role of estrogen therapy in prostate cancer. *Clin Prostate Cancer.* 2002;1:81–89.

11. Glick JH, Wein A, Padavic K, Negendank W, Harris D, Brodovsky H. Tamoxifen in refractory metastatic carcinoma of the prostate. *Cancer Treat Rep.* 1980;64:813–818.

12. Seidenfeld J, Samson DJ, Hasselblad V, et al. Single-therapy androgen suppression in men with advanced prostate cancer: a systemic review and meta-analysis. *Ann Int Med.* 2000;132:566–577.

13. L. Klotz, L. Boccon-Gibod and N.D. Shore, et al. The efficacy and safety of degarelix: a 12-month, comparative, randomized, open-label, parallel-group phase III study in patients with prostate cancer. *BJU Int.* 2008;102:1531–1538.

14. Chodak G, Sharifi R, Kasimis B, Block NL, Macramalla E, Kiennealey GT. Single agent therapy with bicalutamide: a comparison with medical or surgical castration in the treatment of advanced prostate carcinoma. *Urology*. 1995;46: 849–855.

15. See WA, Wirth MP, McLeod DG, et al. Bicalutamide as immediate therapy either alone or as adjuvant to standard care in patients with localized or locally advanced prostate cancer: first analysis of the early prostate cancer program. *J Urol*. 2002;168:429–435.

16. Medicines and Healthcare Products Regulatory Agency (UK), Committee on Safety of Medications. Casodex 150 mg (bicalutamide) no longer indicated for treatment of localised prostate cancer (Dear Health Professional letter). October 28, 2003.

17. Schellhammer PF, Davis JW. An evaluation of bicalutamide in the treatment of prostate cancer. *Clin Prostate Cancer*. 2004;2:213–219.

18. Scher HI, Kelly WK. Flutamide withdrawal syndrome: its impact on clinical trials in hormone-refractory prostate cancer. *J Clin Oncol*. 1993;11:1566–1572.

19. Kassouf W, Tanguay S, Aprikian AG. Nilutamide as second line hormone therapy for prostate cancer after androgen ablation fails. *J Urol*. 2003;169:1742–1744.

20. Joyce R, Fenton MA, Rode P, et al. High dose bicalutamide for androgen independent prostate cancer: effect of prior hormonal therapy. *J Urol*. 1998;159:149–153.

21. Small EJ, Baron AD, Fippin L, Apodaca D, et al. Ketoconazole retains activity in advanced prostate cancer patients with progression after androgen ablation fails. *J Urol*. 1997;157(4): 1204–1207.

22. Tannock I, Gospodarowicz M, Meakin W, Panzarella T, Stewart L, Rider W. Treatment of metastatic prostatic cancer with low-dose prednisone: evaluation of pain and quality of life as pragmatic indicators of response. *J Clin Oncol*. 1989;7:590–597.

23. Osborn JL, Smith DC, Trump DL. Megestrol acetate in the treatment of hormone refractory prostate cancer. *Am J Clin Oncol*. 1997;20:308–310.

24. Crawford ED, Eisenberger MA, McLeod DG, et al. A controlled trial of leuprolide with and without flutamide in prostatic carcinoma. *N Engl J Med*. 1989;321:419–424.

25. Crawford ED, Eisenberger MA, McLeod DG, Wilding G, Blumenstein BA. Comparison of bilateral orchiectomy with or without flutamide for the treatment of patients with stage D2 adenocarcinoma of the prostate: results of NCI intergroup study 0105. *J Urol.* 1997;157(suppl):336.

26. Prostate Cancer Trialists' Collaborative Group. Maximum androgen blockade in advanced prostate cancer: an overview of the randomized trials. *Lancet.* 2000;355:1491–1498.

27. Byar DP, Corle DK. Hormone therapy for prostate cancer: results of the Veterans Administration Cooperative Urologic Research Group studies. *NCI Monogr.* 1988:165–170.

28. The Medical Research Council Prostate Cancer Working Party Investigators Group. Immediate versus deferred treatment for advanced prostatic cancer: initial result of the Medical Research Council Trial. *Br J Urol.* 1997;79:235–246.

29. Bolla M, Gonzalez D, Warde P, et al. Improved survival in patients with locally advanced prostate cancer treated with radiotherapy and goserelin. *N Engl J Med.* 1997;337:295–300.

30. Pilepich MV, Caplan R, Byhardt RW, et al. Phase III trial of androgen suppression using goserelin in unfavorable-prognosis carcinoma of the prostate treated with definitive radiotherapy: report of Radiation Therapy Oncology Group Protocol 85-31. *J Clin Oncol.* 1997;15:1013–1021.

31. Messing EM, Manola J, Sarosdy M, Wilding G, Crawford ED, Trump D. Immediate hormonal therapy compared with observation after radical prostatectomy and pelvic lymphadenectomy in men with node-positive prostate cancer. *N Engl J Med.* 1999;341:1781–1788.

32. Sandford NL, Searle JW, Kerr JF. Successive waves of apoptosis in the rat prostate after repeated withdrawal of testosterone stimulation. *Pathology.* 1984;16:406–410.

33. de Leval J, Boca P, Yousef E, et al. Intermittent versus continuous total androgen blockade in the treatment of patients with advanced hormone-naive prostate cancer: results of a prospective randomized multicenter trial. *Clin Prostate Cancer.* 2002;1:163–171.

34. Rashid MH, Chaudhary UB. Intermittent androgen deprivation therapy for prostate cancer. *Oncologist.* 2004;9:295–301.

35. Higano CS. Side effects of androgen deprivation therapy: monitoring and minimizing toxicity. *Urology.* 2003;61(suppl 1):32–38.

36. Loprinzi CL, Michalak JC, Quella SK, et al. Megestrol acetate for the prevention of hot flashes. *N Engl J Med.* 1994;331:347–352.

37. Melton JL III, Alothman KI, Khosla S, Achenbach SJ, Oberg AL, Zincke H. Fracture risk following bilateral orchiectomy. *J Urol*. 2003;169:1747–1750.

38. Smith MR, McGovern FJ, Zietman AL, et al. Pamidronate to prevent bone loss during androgen-deprivation therapy for prostate cancer. *N Engl J Med*. 2001;345:948–955.

39. Smith MR, Eastham J, Gleason DM, et al. Randomized controlled trial of zoledronic acid to prevent bone loss in men receiving androgen deprivation therapy for nonmetastatic prostate cancer. *J Urol*. 2003;169:2008–2012.

40. Loblaw DA, Mendelson DS, Talcott JA, et al. American Society of Clinical Oncology recommendations for the initial hormonal management of androgen-sensitive metastatic, recurrent, or progressive prostate cancer. *J Clin Oncol*. 2004;22:2927–2941.

41. Nelson WG, De Marzo AM, Isaacs WB. Prostate cancer. *N Engl J Med*. 2003;349:366–381.

42. Shaffer DR, Scher HI. Prostate cancer: a dynamic illness with shifting targets. *Lancet Oncol*. 2003;4:407–414.

43. Feldman BJ, Feldman D. The development of androgen-independent prostate cancer. *Nat Rev Cancer*. 2001;1:34–45.

44. Crawford ED, Tombal B, Miller K, et al. A phase III extension trial with a 1-arm crossover from leuprolide to degarelix: comparison of gonadotropin-releasing hormone agonist and antagonist effect on prostate cancer. *J Urol*. 2011;186:889–897.

45. Scher HI, Beer TM, Higano CS, et al. Antitumour activity of MDV3100 in castration-resistant prostate cancer: a phase 1-2 study. *Lancet*. 2010;375(9724):1437–1446.

46. Rathkoph DE, Danila DC, Slovin S, et al. A first-in-human, open-label, phase I/II safety, pharmacokinetic, and proof-of-concept study of ARN-509 in patients with progressive advanced castration-resistant prostate cancer (CRPC). *J Clin Oncol*. 29: 2011 (suppl; abstr TPS190).

47. Sawyers CL New insights into the prostate cancer genome and therapeutic implications. Proceedings of the prostate cancer foundation annual scientific retreat, Washington DC, 2010.

48. De Bono JS, Logothetis MD, Molina A Abiraterone and increased survival in metastatic prostate cancer. *N Engl J Med*. 2011;21(364): 1995–2005.

49. Agus DB, Stadler WM, Shevrin DH. Safety, efficacy and pharmodynamics of the investigational agent TAK-700 in metatstic castration-resistant prostate cancer (mCRPC): updated data from a Phase I/II study. *J Clin Oncol*. 29: 2011; (suppl; abstr 4531).

50. Klotz L, Schellhammer P, Carroll K A re-assesment of the role of combined androgen blockade for advanced prostate cancer. *BJU International*. 2004;93:1177–1182.

51. Chodak G, Gomella L, Phung de H. Combined androgen blockade in advanced prostate cancer: looking back to move forward. *Clin Genitourin Cancer*. 2007;5(6):371–378.

52. Moul JW, Wu H, Sun L, et al. Early versus delayed hormonal therapy for prostate specific antigen only recurrence of prostate cancer after radical prostatectomy. *J Urol*. 2008;179(5):S53–59.

53. Shaw GL, Wilson P, Cuzick J, et al. International study into the use of intermittent hormone therapy in the treatment of carcinoma of the prostate: a meta-analysis of 1446 patients. *BJU Int*. 2007;99(5):1056–1065.

54. Shore ND, Crawford ED. Intermittent androgen deprivation therapy: redefining the standard of care? *Rev Urol*. 2010 Winter;12(1):1–11.

55. Irani J, Salomon L, Oba R, et al. Efficacy of venlafaxine, medroxyprogesterone acetate and cyproterone acetate for the treatment of vasomotor hot flashes in men taking gonadotropin-releasing hormone analogues for prostate cancer: a double blind, randomized trial. *Lancet Oncol*. 2010;11:147–154.

56. Smith MR, Egerdie B, Hernández Toriz N, et al. Denosumab in men receiving androgen-deprivation therapy for prostate cancer. *N Engl J Med*. 2009;361:745–755.

57. Tombal B, Miller K, Boccon-Gibod L, et al. Additional analysis of the secondary end point of biochemical recurrence rate in a phase 3 trial (CS21) comparing degarelix 80 mg versus leuprolide in prostate cancer patients segmented by baseline characteristics. *Eur Urol*. 2010;57:836–42.

58. Studer UE, Collette I, Whelan P, et al. EORTC Genitourinary Group. Using PSA to guide timing of androgen deprivation in patients with T0–4 N0–2 M0 prostate cancer not suitable for local curative treatment (EORTC 30891), *Eur Urol*. 2008; 53: 941–949.

Treatment of Castrate-Resistant Prostate Cancer (CRPC)

■ Introduction

Androgen suppressive therapy (AST), while offering effective palliation and perhaps some improvement in survival for patients with advanced prostate cancer, clearly is not curative. All men treated with AST will eventually demonstrate progression of disease unless they die of other causes. The medium time to progression is said to be anywhere between 14 and 30 months, with a great deal of variability noted in clinical practice. Survival after the development of androgen independence is said to be dismal.[1] Yet, many of these men maintain a performance status that allows and perhaps encourages further anticancer treatment. Until very recently, treatment with chemotherapy had not shown any survival benefit. Recent work, to be discussed in this chapter, suggests that a more optimistic view is warranted. Additionally, new targeted therapies and treatment aimed at improving the immune response to prostate cancer have become available. However, the decision to start chemotherapy, like all other therapeutic decisions in prostate cancer, should not be a reflexive one. Instead, it should be the result of an honest discussion between the physician and the patient regarding the advantages and disadvantages of the proposed treatment.

Many issues involving chemotherapy for CRPC remain unsettled. How is the state defined? What prognostic factors predict response? How is response measured? The measurement of PSA levels has traditionally been used as a marker of response and prognosis. Cross-sectional imaging is accurate for measuring some soft tissue lesions, but evaluation of response in bone by any modality remains problematic. The measure of circulating tumor cells is being studied as a more accurate indicator of response and prognosis.[41]

This section deals with the overall management of CRPC. It starts with current chemotherapy options, touches on experimental and novel therapies, and includes adjunctive measures.

■ Definition of Castrate-Resistant State

■ In general, CRPC implies objective progression of the disease while the patient is in the castrate state. Most published criteria were developed for the purpose of defining eligibility for clinical trials in CRPC. The following criteria seem reasonable in clinical practice:

  * Serum testosterone levels less than 30 ng/ml AND one of the following:

    ■ Increase in measurable soft tissue or visceral disease on either CT, MRI, or other radiographic imaging

    ■ Development of new metastatic lesions on radio-nuclide bone scanning (worsening of previously known abnormal areas is not sufficient, as bone repair in response to treatment may be confused with progression)

    ■ Consecutively increasing levels of PSA at least 2 weeks apart

■ Measurement of circulating tumor cells (CTC) has recently come into use to follow response to therapy.[42] At the time of this writing, CTCs have not been used to determine castrate resistance.

■ Chemotherapy

Until 2004, advanced prostate cancer was felt to be a chemotherapy-resistant disease. A review of chemotherapy trials by Yagoda et al.[2] in 1993 failed to reveal any single-agent or combination regimen producing objective response rates of more than 10% or resulting in improved survival. It should be kept in mind that criteria for response, particularly in the pre-PSA era, varied greatly. It is possible that the results of treatment were either exaggerated or underappreciated. With various endpoints being used, several new agents that are active alone or in combination have been identified since then. However, it was not until 2004 that an effect on survival was shown for chemotherapy with docetaxel (see Docetaxel Based Therapy).

- Special toxicity considerations
  - Patients with advanced prostate cancer present unique challenges with regard to their ability to tolerate chemotherapy because of:
    - Age
    - Comorbidities
    - Impaired bone marrow reserve secondary to prior radiotherapy and/or bone marrow metastases
    - Renal dysfunction secondary to obstruction
    - Potential for adverse drug interaction due to the use of multiple medications
    - Poor performance status
  - These factors should be considered and appropriate dose reduction should be applied, when necessary, in using the regimens described in this chapter.
- Chemotherapy prognostic factors
  - In order to stratify patients entering clinical trials, several groups have conducted multivariate analyses to learn which factors predict survival.[3,4]
  - Factors found to influence survival:
    - Karnofsky Performance Status (KPS)
    - Gleason score
    - Hemoglobin level
    - Presence or absence of visceral disease
    - Alkaline phosphatase level
    - Serum albumin level
    - Serum LDH level

■ Historical Background

Single Agents

- Estramustine phosphate
  - An oral agent consisting of estradiol linked to nitrogen mustard
  - Initially developed with the idea that the estrogen moiety would target prostate cancer cells, bringing the cytotoxic agent into the cell, where it would be cleaved off and result in cell death—the Trojan horse strategy

- Mode of action currently thought to be based on binding to microtubule-associated proteins, with mitosis inhibition resulting from promotion of microtubule disassembly.[5]
- Single-agent response rates ranging from 14% to 67% reported in early literature.[1,6]
- Subsequent trials comparing estramustine with anti-androgens, placebo, or chemotherapy failed to show a survival advantage or palliative benefits.[7–9]
- Toxicity
  - Nausea and vomiting
  - Elevated liver enzymes (more common with intravenous preparations)
  - Thromboembolic events
    - Most clinicians administer prophylactic low-dose or full-dose warfarin to patients on estramustine.
  - Gynecomastia
  - Impotence
  - Myelosuppression
- Dose (single agent)
  - 10 mg/kg/day in three divided doses
  - Supplied as a 140-mg capsule
- Estramustine should be taken on an empty stomach.
  - Milk, dairy products, and other calcium-rich foods should be avoided.
- Clinical use
  - Estramustine is rarely used as single-agent therapy in current practice.
  - It is more commonly used in combination with tubulin binding agents, such as vinca alkaloids or taxanes, but the value of adding estramustine to other chemotherapy agents is currently being questioned.
- Cyclophosphamide
  - An oral (or intravenous) alkylating agent long considered active in prostate cancer
  - Single-agent activity 30%[10]

- Dose
  - 100–150 mg/day for 21 out of 28 days
- Toxicity
  - Nausea and vomiting
  - Alopecia
  - Leukopenia
- Clinical use
  - Oral cyclophosphamide is generally used in heavily pretreated patients for whom few options beyond comfort care are available.
- Metronomic cyclophosphamide
  - Another way of administering cyclophosphamide was reported by Glode et al.[11] Low-dose cyclophosphamide (50 mg/day every morning) was combined with low-dose dexamethasone (1 mg at night) in what was termed metronomic therapy.
  - 68% of patients experienced a PSA response, leading the author to suggest this approach as salvage therapy.
- Etoposide
  - A topoisomerase II inhibitor that can be given orally or intravenously
  - Dose (single agent)
    - 50 mg/m^2 (50–100 mg) orally once daily for 21 out of 28 days
  - Toxicity
    - Alopecia
    - Anorexia
    - Acute hypersensitivity reaction (rare when oral etoposide is used)
    - Myelosuppression
  - Clinical use
    - Minimally active as a single agent[12] but used in combination regimens, particularly for high-grade, neuroendocrine, or small cell prostate cancers

Combination Chemotherapy

▪ Doxorubicin and ketoconazole

* Use of doxorubicin, an intravenous anthracycline, in combination is based on a single-agent trial demonstrating improved symptom control compared with prednisone.[13]
* Doxorubicin is more commonly used in combination with ketoconazole.
  ▪ Millikan et al.[14] reported better PSA control (36% vs. 31%) but more toxicity with the combination of ketoconazole and doxorubicin compared with ketoconazole alone.
  ▪ Culine et al[15] reported a 50% PSA response rate and a 45% objective response rate, but toxicity caused 20% of patients to discontinue treatment.
* Dose
  ▪ Doxorubicin: 20 mg/m^2 IV once weekly
  ▪ Ketoconazole: 200 mg three times per day
* Toxicity
  ▪ Nausea and vomiting
  ▪ Alopecia
  ▪ Cardiotoxicity
  ▪ Myelosuppression
* Clinical use
  ▪ Significant toxicity and the emergence of more effective chemotherapy regimens limit usefulness of this regimen.

▪ Vinblastine and estramustine

* Vinblastine is a plant (vinca) alkaloid that inhibits mitosis through tubulin binding.
* Activity
  ▪ PSA response rates (> 50% decrease in PSA level) of 54% and 61%, and objective response rates in measurable disease of 12–20%, were seen in Phase II trials conducted by Hudes et al[16] and Seidman et al.[17]
    * Significant palliative effects were also seen. Median duration of response was 7 months in the Seidman trial.

- In a randomized trial comparing vinblastine alone with vinblastine plus estramustine, a trend for improved survival that was not statistically significant was noted for the combination.[18]
- There was a statistically significant advantage for the combination in time to progression and PSA response.
  - Dose schedule
    - Vinblastine: 4 mg/m^2 IV once weekly for 6 weeks
    - Estramustine: 600 mg/m^2 daily for 42 days
    - Recycle every 56 days
  - Toxicity
    - Nausea and vomiting
    - Neuropathy
    - Edema
    - Myelosuppression
    - Toxicity and the availability of better systemic therapies limit the usefulness of this regimen.
- Mitoxantrone and prednisone
  - This regimen was approved for treatment of symptomatic CRPC based on a study by Tannock et al.[19] in which relief of pain was the primary endpoint.
    - In this study, 161 patients with pain were randomized to receive either prednisone alone or prednisone plus mitoxantrone. Mitoxantrone plus prednisone (MP) was superior to prednisone alone in the achievement of pain control (29% vs. 12%) and median duration of palliation (43 weeks vs. 18 weeks).
    - No difference in overall survival was noted, and objective responses were not reported.
    - Effective palliation with this regimen was not confirmed in a second trial conducted by Kantoff et al.,[20] but differences in methodology and patient characteristics make drawing conclusions difficult.
  - Dose schedule
    - Mitoxantrone: 12 mg/m^2 IV once every 3 weeks
    - Prednisone: 5 mg orally twice daily

- Toxicity
  - Minimal nausea and vomiting
  - Minimal alopecia
  - Myelosuppression
  - Cardiotoxicity
- Clinical use
  - This is a well-tolerated regimen aimed primarily at symptom (pain) relief.
  - In trials described later, mitoxantrone + prednisone (M + P) was found to be inferior to docetaxel-based regimens, making M + P a second- or third-line approach.
  - This regimen could also be considered for symptomatic patients who are unable to tolerate more aggressive approaches.

Taxane-Based Regimens

- The taxanes (paclitaxel and docetaxel) inhibit mitosis by binding to and interfering with the depolymerization of tubulin, causing arrest in the G2M phase of the cell cycle, leading to apoptosis.
- Docetaxel may also promote apoptosis by inducing phosphorylation of bcl-2, resulting in loss of its antiapoptotic function.[21]
- Pretreatment with corticosteroids and histamine blockers to prevent acute hypersensitivity reactions is required with these agents.
- None of the paclitaxel-based or nontaxane combinations have been shown to improve survival.
- Two studies involving docetaxel presented at the 2004 annual meeting of the American Society of Clinical Oncology (ASCO) were the first to demonstrate a survival benefit for any cytotoxic chemotherapy in this disease.
  - As a result, docetaxel was approved for the treatment of hormone-refractory prostate cancer, and its use has superseded that of other agents as first-line therapy in this setting.

- Paclitaxel-based therapy
  - The inclusion of paclitaxel in combination therapy for CPMC is based on single-agent trials demonstrating efficacy.
    - Although little activity and significant toxicity resulted when paclitaxel was given as a 24-hour continuous infusion weekly,[22] Trivedi[23] treated 18 patients with weekly 1-hour infusions of pactlitaxel and noted a 39% PSA response rate. Objective responses were observed in patients with measurable disease.
  - Most trials combined a taxane with estramustine in a combined antimicrotubule strategy.
  - Paclitaxel and estramustine
    - A variety of trials employing paclitaxel by continuous infusion, or by 1-hour weekly infusion with estramustine given either on a daily basis or 3–5 days per week, has been reported.
      - Summarized in a review by Petrylak,[24] these trials revealed PSA response rates of between 38% and 67% and objective response rates of 27–46%. In general, toxicities included neuropathy, nausea and vomiting, and thromboembolic events.
  - Paclitaxel + Carboplatin + Estramustine
    - Kelly et al.,[25] in a Phase II trial involving 56 patients, reported a highly active regimen that added carboplatin to paclitaxel and estramustine.
      - Treatment schedule*
        - Estramustine: 10 mg/kg PO daily for 5 days starting 2 days before each weekly paclitaxel dose
        - Paclitaxel: 60–100 mg/m^2 IV over 1 hour once weekly
        - Carboplatin: AUC = 5 or 6 IV once every 4 weeks
          - *Off study, a reasonable starting dose of weekly paclitaxel is 80 mg/m^2, with estramustine given for only 3–5 days each week.
          - The paclitaxel is delivered on the middle day (day 2 or 3) of the estramustine regimen.

- Full- or low-dose warfarin should strongly be considered, and pretreatment with steroids and histamine blockers is strongly recommended.
- Activity
  - PSA response rate of 67%
  - Response rate in measurable disease of 45%, including 2/33 (6%) complete responders
- Toxicity
  - Thromboembolic events
  - Hyperglycemia (probably due to pretreatment corticosteroids)
  - Hypophosphatemia
  - Significant myelosuppression and neuropathy were not seen.
- Clinical use
  - Carboplatin-containing regimens have not been tested in large Phase 3 trial.
  - The combination of carboplatin and paclitaxel has been successfully used in the MSKCC group as second- or third-line chemotherapy after docetaxel.
    - Starting doses are carboplatinum AUC 5 or 6 q 4 weeks and paclitaxel 80 mg/m^2 weekly for 3 or 4 weeks.
    - Alternately, for heavily treated patients or those with poor KPS the carboplatinum can be given once weekly at a targeted AUC of 1–1.5.

■ Current Chemotherapy

- Docetaxel is the standard first-line chemotherapy regimen.
- Studies of single-agent docetaxel, given either weekly at 35–36 mg/m^2 or every 21 days at 75 mg/m^2, yielded PSA response rates of 38–58% and response rates in measurable disease of 17–40%.[24]
- In general, toxicities of docetaxel include myelosuppression, nail and skin changes, fatigue, and less commonly, pulmonary toxicity.

- When docetaxel was given every 3 weeks with intermittent estramustine in two Phase I trials, response rates of 63–82% were observed.[26,27]
- It was not until 2004, when the results of two studies, SWOG 99-16 and TAX 327, were presented at the annual ASCO meeting, that a survival benefit was shown for docetaxel-based chemotherapy.
  - SWOG 99-16[28]
    - A randomized Phase III trial looking primarily at survival that involved 770 men with castrate resistant prostate cancer (AIPC) compared docetaxel + estramustine with mitoxantrone + prednisone
    - Treatment schedule
      - **Arm A**
        - Docetaxel: 60 mg/m^2 IV on day 2
        - Estramustine: 280 mg PO three times daily for 5 days
        - Recycle every 21 days
      - **Arm B**
        - Mitoxantrone: 12 mg/m^2 IV every 21 days
        - Prednisone: 5 mg PO daily
      - *Note*: Dose escalation of docetaxel to 70 mg/m^2 and of mitoxantrone to 14 mg/m^2 was allowed if no grade 3–4 toxicities were seen after cycle 1.
      - Patients receiving docetaxel received pretreatment dexamethasone 20 mg PO three times in the 24 hours preceding chemotherapy.
        - Patients receiving estramustine, who were enrolled later in the study, were given warfarin 2 mg once daily and aspirin 325 mg once daily.
      - Results
        - There was a statistically significant improvement in survival (17.5 months vs. 15.6 months, log rank, p = .02) in favor of the docetaxel + estramustine arm as well as a shorter time to progression (p = < .0001).
        - A significant difference in PSA response (50% vs 27%, p < .001) was also seen in the docetaxel + estramustine arm.

- Objective response in measurable disease was 17% for the docetaxel + estramustine arm versus 11% for mitoxantrone + prednisone (p = .15).
- Overall, this translated into a 27% improvement in PFS and a 20% predicted decrease in death for the docetaxel + estramustine arm.
  - Toxicity
    - Higher GI and cardiovascular toxicity (grade 3–4, 54%) was seen in the docetaxel + estramustine arm compared with 34% in the mitoxantrone + prednisone arm, but there was no difference in deaths due to toxicity or withdrawal from study because of toxicity.
- TAX 327[29]
  - A randomized phase III trial involving 1,006 men with AIPC that compared weekly docetaxel + prednisone, q 3-week docetaxel + prednisone, and q 3-week mitoxantrone + prednisone
  - The primary endpoint was survival, with secondary endpoints including PSA response, pain response, and toxicity.
  - Treatment schedule
    - **Arm A**
      - Docetaxel: 75 mg/m^2 IV q 3 weeks
      - Prednisone: 5 mg PO twice daily
    - **Arm B**
      - Docetaxel: 30 mg/m^2 IV weekly for 5 weeks out of 6
      - Prednisone: 5 mg PO twice daily
    - **Arm C**
      - Mitoxantrone: 12 mg/m^2 IV q 3 weeks
      - Prednisone: 5 mg PO twice daily
    - Patients were treated for 30 weeks.
    - All patients on docetaxel received dexamethasone prior to chemotherapy.

- Results
  - Docetaxel + prednisone, when given every 3 weeks but not when given weekly, was superior to mitoxantrone + prednisone in overall survival (18.9 months vs. 16.5 months, p = .009), pain response (35% vs. 22%, p = .01), and PSA response (45% vs. 32%, p = .0005).
- Toxicity
  - There was more grade 3–4 neutropenia in the q 3-week docetaxel arm (32%) compared with the weekly docetaxel (1.5%) and the q 3-week mitoxantrone (21.7%) arms.
  - Although neutropenic fever and neutropenic infections were more common in the q 3-week docetaxel arm, no deaths from sepsis were reported.
  - Nonhematologic toxicity was similar in all three arms, with the exception of increased neurosensory symptoms, nail changes, and eye changes in the docetaxel arms.
  - Survival data for Tax 327 was updated in 2008[43]
    - With 310 additional deaths, the survival advantage for q 3-week docetaxel plus daily prednisone over mitoxantrone plus prednisone persisted.
    - Median survival for the docetaxel arm was 19.2 months (95% CI of 17.5–21.3 months) vs. 16.3 months (95% CI of 14.3–17.9 months) for the mitoxantrone prednisone arm; p = 0.004.
  - Conclusions
    - SWOG 99-16 and TAX 327 are well-powered randomized trials that seem to establish q 3-week docetaxel at 75 mg/m^2 plus prednisone 10 mg/day plus prednisone as the preferred first-line chemotherapy for symptomatic hormone-refractory prostate cancer. The dose of docetaxel should be reduced, or the drug should not be given at all to patients with significant liver dysfunction depending on the degree of liver dysfunction.

- The role of estramustine in taxane-based combinations
  - The increased risk of GI toxicity and thromboembolic events mandates serious assessment of the value of adding estramustine to docetaxel.
  - Increased PSA response and time to progression were reported by Hudes et al.[18] when estramustine was added to vinblastine compared with vinblastine alone.
  - Similar findings favoring the addition of estramustine to paclitaxel compared with paclitaxel alone were reported by Berry et al.,[30] but neither study demonstrated a survival advantage.
  - Although no direct comparison can be made between SWOG 99-16 (docetaxel + estramustine) and TAX 327 (docetaxel + prednisone), the overall survival curves were similar.
  - At this time, the value of adding estramustine to taxane-based regimens remains unclear.
- Docetaxel practical considerations
- On the basis of these two trials, docetaxel 75 mg/m^2 every 3 weeks plus prednisone 5 mg orally twice daily has become the standard first-line chemotherapy regimen for patients with castrate-resistant prostate cancer.
- Toxicity is acceptable.
  - Fatigue is common during the first week after docetaxel.
  - Nausea and vomiting are rare.
  - Tearing, hair loss, and nail changes are common.
  - Corticosteroids plus histamine (H1 and H2) blockers are routinely given to prevent acute hypersensitivity reactions (HSR).
    - Reactions are usually manifested by severe back pain.
      - Shortness of breath and IGE-mediated reactions are rare.
    - HSRs are frequently managed by stopping the infusion, giving extra doses of steroid or antihistamines, and restarting the infusion at a slower rate.
    - Patients who have severe or anaphylactic reactions should probably not receive further docetaxel.

- Most patients receiving q 3-week docetaxel do not need prophylactic colony–stimulating factors such as pegfilgrastim.
  - But, patients with poor marrow reserve or those with suboptimal performance status should be considered for prophylactic pegfilgrastim.
    - Another option for such patients would be weekly docetaxel ($25–30$ mg/m^2) 3 weeks out of 4 or another regimen such as mitoxantrone plus prednisone.
- Edema and diarrhea can occur.

Cabazitaxel

- Standard second-line chemotherapy for patients who progress through docetaxel.
- Cabazitaxel is a tubulin-binding taxane with activity in patients who fail docetaxel.
- de Bono et al.[44] randomized 755 men with castration-resistant prostate cancer who progressed through docetaxel chemotherapy to:
  - Mitoxantrone 12 mg/m^2 once every 3 weeks + prednisone versus
  - Cabazitaxel 25 mg/m^2 once every 3 weeks + prednisone
    - Patients receiving cabazitaxel received single doses of dexamethasone (8 mg), an H1 blocker, and an H2 (histamine) blocker immediately before treatment.
  - Overall survival was the primary endpoint.
    - Progression-free survival and safety were secondary endpoints
  - Results
    - Median survival was 15.1 months (95% CI of 14.1–16.3) for the cabazitaxel arm and 12.7 months (95% CI of 11.6–13.7) for the mitoxantrone arm.
    - Hazard ratio for death for men treated with cabazitaxel over those treated with mitoxantrone was 0.70 (95% CI of 0.59–0.83); $p < 0.0001$
    - Median progression-free survival was 2.8 months (95% CI of 2.4–3.0) in the cabazitaxel arm versus 1.4 months (95% CI of 1.4–1.7).
    - Hazard ratio for progression favored cabazitaxel HR 0.74 (95% CI of 0.64–0.86); $p < 0.0001$

- Toxicity in the cabazitaxel arm:
  - 82% had grade 3 or higher neutropenia but only 8% had febrile neutropenia.
  - 6% had diarrhea.
- Comments on cabazitaxel:
  - On the basis of this trial, cabazitaxel is considered standard second-line chemotherapy for patients with castrate-resistant prostate cancer who have progressed through docetaxel.
  - Pegfilgrastim should be considered for high-risk patients because of the high incidence of neutropenia.

Investigational Agents

A large number of investigational agents are currently in various stages of development. A complete review is beyond the scope of this handbook. One drug merits comment because of promising data reported at the Genitourinary Cancers Symposium 2011[45]:

- Cabozantinib (XL 184)
  (Not to be confused with Cabazitaxel!)
  - Targets MET and VEGF 2 receptors, signaling pathways involved in osteoblast and osteoclast function
    - 72 patients with CRPC and measurable disease with or without bone metastases who had no disease progression after no more than one prior chemotherapy regimen
    - XL given orally for 12 weeks
    - Primary endpoint is objective response at 12 weeks.
    - Results at 12 weeks
      - 24 patients were evaluable at the time of the report.
      - 5 out of 24 (21%) had partial (> 30% reduction in measurable disease) response.
      - 6 out of 24 (25%) had 50% reduction in PSA.
      - 13 out of 15 (87%) had either complete or partial resolution of lesions on bone scan.
      - 11 out of 15 patients with bone pain were noted to have less pain.
      - Markers of bone turnover and serum alkaline phosphatase declined by 66% and 63% respectively.

- Toxicity
  - Grade 3 or higher fatigue: 10%
  - Grade 3 or higher diarrhea: 3%
  - Grade 3 or higher elevations of AST: 3%
- *Comment*: Cabozantinib (XL 184) appears to be a very active agent particularly for bone metastases. The results of the completed trial are eagerly awaited.

Antiangiogenic Therapy

- Bevacizumab: when combined with docetaxel and prednisone did not improve survival compared with docetaxel and prednisone alone. In fact, survival was worse.[46]
- Other VEGF inhibitors or kinase inhibitors under investigation include
  - Aflibercept
  - Sunitinib
  - Lenalidomide
- A more detailed review of developing therapies was published by Aggarwal and Ryan.[47]

■ Chemotherapy for High-Grade and Unusual Histology Prostate Cancer

- Even patients with high-grade (Gleason scores of 8–10), poorly differentiated cancers may respond to hormone therapy, although the duration of response to hormones is typically short.
- When chemotherapy is needed, docetaxel remains the first drug of choice. Some clinicians prefer carboplatin-based regimens.
- Patients with pure small cell histology should be treated with cisplatin plus etoposide. Carboplatin may be used in place of cisplatin for patients with impaired renal function or those who may otherwise not tolerate cisplatin.
  - AST is sometimes used in addition to chemotherapy
- Lymphomas, sarcomas, and transitional cell carcinomas should be treated with standard regimens for those histologies.
  - Androgen-suppressive therapy is not useful in these histologic forms.

■ Immunotherapy of Castrate-Resistant Prostate Cancer

- ▓ Sipuleucel-T was approved for the treatment of metastatic castrate-resistant prostate cancer in 2010 based on a the Phase 3 Immunotherapy Prostate AdenoCarcinoma Treatment (IMPACT) trial.
- ▓ This program involves a series of steps aimed at stimulating the immune system to attack prostate cancer cells.
  - Patients undergo three leukapheresis episodes 2 weeks apart.
  - At a processing lab, the mononuclear antigen-presenting cells are incubated with a GM-CSF-Prostatic Acid Phosphatase fusion protein known as PA2024.
  - Three days after collection, the patient receives these CD 54 positive cells by infusion after premedication with acetaminophen and antihistamines.
- ▓ Two prior randomized, placebo-controlled trials failed to meet the primary endpoint, which was time to disease progression.
  - One of the trials showed a trend toward improved survival.
  - The other showed a statistically significant improvement in survival for sipuleucel-T over placebo; HR 0.59 (95% CI of 0.39–0.88; p = 0.01).
  - Approval by the FDA was withheld because the primary endpoint was not reached.
- ▓ The IMPACT trial[48] was a double-blind, placebo-controlled multicenter randomization of 512 patients to either sipuleucel-T or placebo in a 2:1 ratio.
  - Patients assigned to the placebo arm underwent leukapheresis as described above, but were reinfused with antigen-presenting cells that had not been incubated with PA2024 (the GMCSF-acid phosphatase fusion protein).
- ▓ Eligibility
  - Metastatic CRPC
  - Either asymptomatic or minimally symptomatic

- Initially only patients with Gleason scores of 7 or less were included.
  - Eligibility later broadened to include all Gleason scores.
- No more than two prior chemotherapy regimens and no chemotherapy in 3 months
- Patients remained on androgen suppression and bisphosphonates.
- Primary endpoint was survival adjusted for baseline PSA levels.
- Results
  - There was a 22% reduction in the risk of death in the sipuleucel-T group compared with placebo; HR 0.78 (95% CI of 0.61–0.98; p = 0.03).
  - This translates to a 4.1-month increase in survival (25.8 months vs 21.7 months).
  - At 36 months, the probability of survival was 31.7% for the sipuleucel group and 23% in the placebo group.
  - There was no difference in time to disease progression: 3.6 months in the sipuleucel-T group versus 3.6 months in the placebo group.
  - PSA levels decreased by more than 50% in 8 of 311 (2.6%) in the treatment arm and 2 of 153 (1.3%) of patients in the placebo arm.
  - One patient receiving sipuleucel-T had an objective response.
  - Toxicity was generally mild (< Grade 3) and transient in the treatment group
    - Virtually all patients had grade 1–2 toxicity of some type and approximately one-third had grade 3 or higher toxicity.
    - Fever: 29.3 %
    - Chills: 54.1%
    - Back pain: 34.3%
    - Nausea: 28.1%
    - Fatigue : 39.1%
    - Miscellaneous, grade < 3: 20% or less

- Comment on Sipuleucel-T:
  - The results of the IMPACT trial showed a survival benefit in the absence of objective improvement or delay in time to progression. But, it is an option for minimally or asymptomatic patients with castrate-resistant prostate cancer, Therapy with sipuleucel-T is covered by Medicare, which essentially defrays the large cost of the treatment. Studies examining the role of sipuleucel-T in earlier stages of prostate cancer, where a smaller tumor burden is more likely to respond to immunomodulationt, are either underway or in planning.
    - Other immunotherapeutic agents under investigation[49]:
      - Ipilimumab: an anticytotoxic T-lymphocyte–associated antigen-4 (CTLA-4) antibody
      - GVAX: a combination of LNCap and PC-3 prostate cancer cell lines modified with the GM-CSF gene.
      - PROSTVAC: fowlpox and vaccinia vectors with costimulatory genes

Additional Approaches to Patients with CRPC

- The management of CRPC certainly involves more than just chemotherapy. A separate handbook in this series addresses palliative care, including pain control. The management of specific complications of advanced prostate cancer is the subject of another chapter. This section deals with other modalities commonly employed in patients with AIPC.

The Management of Skeletal Metastases

- Skeletal metastases, very common in patients with CRPC, are responsible for a large part of the morbidity of this disease. Severe pain, or neurologic deficits due to spinal cord compression or direct extension of bone metastases (e.g., base of skull) can result in immobilization and loss of higher function, resulting in a major negative effect on quality-of-life and probably survival.

- ▣ Because most bone metastases from prostate cancer are blastic rather than lytic, pathologic fractures are rare—at least in weight-bearing or long bones. Skeletal metastases in general respond to hormone therapy and occasionally to chemotherapy as well.
- ▣ However, as patients with AIPC live longer because of improved treatment, management options for symptomatic skeletal metastases in patients with castration-resistant disease become critically important.
  - ◦ Bisphosphonates
    - ▣ Bisphosphonates are synthetic compounds, similar to pyrophosphate, that inhibit normal and pathologic bone resorption in a variety of ways.[31] They have been shown to reduce skeletal complications in a variety of other cancers. Even though prostate cancer metastases are typically blastic and bisphosphonates primarily inhibit osteoclasts, bisphosphonates are effective in patients with bone metastases from prostate cancer.
    - ▣ A 24-month follow-up of a large randomized, placebo-controlled trial was reported in 2004[32]:
      - ◦ Intervention
        - ▣ Zoledronic acid 4 mg or 8 mg IV over 15 minutes every 3 weeks versus placebo (because of excess renal toxicity, the 8-mg dose is not recommended and in fact doses less than 4 mg are safer in patients with renal insufficiency). Online calculators are available for dosing zoledronic acid in patient with decreased renal function.
      - ◦ Endpoints
        - ▣ Primary
          - ◦ Proportion of patients having at least one skeletal-related event (SRE)
          - ◦ Pathologic fracture
          - ◦ Spinal cord compression
          - ◦ Need for surgery or radiotherapy for a bone metastasis
          - ◦ Change in systemic antineoplastic therapy in order to treat bone pain

- Secondary
  - Time to first SRE
  - Annual incidence of SREs
  - Mean change from baseline in Brief Pain Inventory score
- Results
  - 38% of patients in the zoledronic acid group versus 49% in the placebo group had a single SRE (p = .028)
  - Annual incidence of SREs was 0.77 for the zoledronic acid group versus 1.47 for the placebo group (p = .28).
  - Median time to first SRE was 488 days for the zoledronic acid group versus 321 days for the control group (p = .009).
  - Significant improvement in Brief Pain Inventory scores was noted for the zoledronic acid group compared with the placebo group.
- Toxicity
  - Mild to moderate fatigue, fever, and myalgias were more common in the zoledronic acid group.
  - Although not commented upon in this report, severe hypocalcemia, pain flare, and radiation recall effects have been seen by this author.
  - Atrial fibrillation and unexpected fractures of long bones have been reported anecdotally
  - Osteonecrosis of the jaw was reported in 2004 in a retrospective review of patients receiving this drug for breast cancer or myeloma.[33] Careful oral examination is suggested prior to institution of zoledronic acid therapy. Any needed dental extractions should be completed prior to therapy and should be avoided during therapy.
  - The exact rate of jaw osteonecrosis in patients with prostate cancer receiving bisphosphonates is not known.

- Denosumab
  - A monoclonal antibody against the receptor activator of nuclear factor $-\kappa\beta$ ligand (RANKL)
  - A phase 3 randomized controlled trial comparing denosumab 120 mg subcutaneously versus zoledronic acid 4 mg intravenously both given every 4 weeks was reported at ASCO 2010.[50] And fully published in 2011.[51]
    - 1901 patients with CRPC and at least one bone metastasis were entered.
    - All patients had failed at least one hormonal therapy.
    - No prior bisphosphonates for bone metastases were allowed.
    - Patients with creatinine clearances of less than 0.5 mL/s were excluded.
    - All patients received vitamin D at least 500 units and calcium at least 500 mg daily.
    - Primary endpoint was time to first skeletal-related event (SRE)
      - Pathologic fracture
      - Malignant spinal cord compression
      - Institution of palliative RT or surgery to bone
  - Results
    - Denosumab delayed first on study SRE 20.7 months vs. 17.1 months for zoledronic acid
    - A difference of 18%
    - HR 0.82 (95% CI of 0.71–0.95; p = 0.008)
    - There was no difference in overall survival or time to progression
    - Denosumab resulted in greater suppression of markers of bone turnover compared to zoledronic acid
  - Toxicity
    - Hypocalcemia occurred in 13% of patients receiving denosumab and 6% of patients receiving zoledronic acid (p < 0.0001)
    - Jaw osteonecrosis was more common in the denosumab arm (2% vs. 1% p = 0.09)

- Other toxicities were generally similar in both groups
  - Anemia
  - Back pain
  - Fatigue
  - Osteonecrosis of the jaw
- At these doses severe (grade 3 and 4) hypocalcemia and hypophosphatemia have been observed (personal communication with Michael M. Morris, MD, October 2011). Guidelines for using this agent are evolving. Patients should be given calcium and vitamin D replacement. The role of serum calcium, phosphorous, and vitamin D levels before and during treatment with denosumab is not yet defined. The drug should either not be used at all or used with great caution in patients with a glomerular filtration rate of less than 30 ml/min.
- Conclusion
  - The evidence suggests that denosumab is superior to zoledronic acid in in preventing skeletal-related events in patients with castration-resistant prostate cancer and bone metastases.
  - Denosumab may be useful in preventing osteoporosis in patients on androgen-suppressive therapy (see Chapter 8).
  - Dose reduction for renal insufficiency is needed for zoledronic acid. The safety of denosumab in patients with severe renal insufficiency is not established and this drug should be used with great caution or not at all in such patients.
  - Although the study cited above used a q 3-week dose of zoledronic acid, the optimal frequency is not yet determined.
  - The use of zoledronic acid in the noncastrate-resistant population and in men without bone metastases is not supported by evidence.
  - Osteonecrosis of the jaw is a problem with both zoledronic acid and denosumab.
  - Vitamin D and calcium supplementation should continue as described in Chapter 8.

■ Palliative EBRT

■ In general, 80% of patients with painful skeletal metastases (from various primary sites) experience relief of pain with EBRT.[34]
  • Treatment course
    ■ Standard treatment is usually delivered in 5–10 fractions.
    ■ Data from 2003 suggest a single fraction may be equally effective and less costly.[35] This approach should be strongly considered for patients who might otherwise require prolonged hospital stays to complete radiotherapy.
  • Toxicity
    ■ Palliative EBRT to skeletal metastases is generally well tolerated.
    ■ Fatigue and myelosuppression are usually the only side effects observed.
    ■ Patients often need to be reassured that nausea and vomiting are rare in this setting.
    ■ However, significant GI toxicity, including diarrhea and even ileus, can occur when the small bowel is included in the radiation field. These side effects are more common when radiotherapy is delivered to pelvic bones or the pelvic cavity.
    ■ Radiotherapy can be given safely with AST.
    ■ Hypofractionated techniques requiring fewer fractions may decrease the inconvenience of multiple daily fractions and reduce hospital stay for those patients requiring inpatient therapy.
  • Limitations
    ■ Expense
    ■ Myelosuppression
    ■ Generally requires interruption of chemotherapy
    ■ Inconvenience when multiple fractions or multiple courses needed
    ■ Patients with CRPC typically have multiple metastatic sites that are painful. Further courses of radiotherapy may not be feasible because of cumulative bone marrow toxicity, concern about overlapping

fields, and the attainment of maximally tolerated dose at a particular site. For these patients, systemic approaches with either chemotherapy or a radiopharmaceutical should be considered, in addition to the usual pain control measures.

- In practice, the cause of an individual's pain and the specific site responsible for it may be difficult to discern.

- Conclusion
  - Palliative EBRT should be considered in the treatment of:
    - Painful bone metastases
    - Neurologic complications, such as spinal cord compression or base of skull involvement
    - Bulky local prostate masses causing pain, obstruction, or bleeding, particularly in patients whose cancer is chemotherapy resistant
  - Soft-tissue metastases at other sites are best treated with AST or chemotherapy.

■ Systemic Radiopharmaceuticals

- The diffuse nature of skeletal metastases in prostate cancer limits the usefulness of EBRT as a palliative maneuver. It is not uncommon to require a course of EBRT to a new site just as, or even before, a current one is completed.

- Chasing one's tail, so to speak, in order to palliate more than two or three sites in a short time frame is rarely productive.

- Systemic therapy with bone-seeking radiopharmaceuticals offers another option in the management of pain due to multiple metastatic skeletal sites. Although none of the currently approved agents have improved survival, significant palliation can be seen even without response that is measured by PSA level decline or change in imaging.

- Currently approved agents[36]
  - Although other systemic radiopharmaceuticals are available or are under investigation, the following two described are the most commonly used in the United States:
    - Strontium chloride 89
      - Beta-emitter similar to calcium in affinity for bone
      - 50.5-day half-life at metastatic sites but much shorter in normal bone[37]
      - Usual dose of 4 mCi
      - Preferential accumulation in bone metastases
      - Improvement in pain in 60–80% of patients
      - Onset of pain relief in 7–21 days
      - Mean duration of pain relief of 6 months
      - Retreatment interval of 90 days because of delayed nadir
    - Samarium 153 ethylene diamine tetramethylene phosphate
      - Combined beta- and gamma-emitter
      - 2-day half-life
      - Usual dose of 0.5–1 mCi/kg
        - Patients with impaired marrow reserve or very poor performance status should probably receive 0.5 mCi/kg rather than 1 mCi/Kg.
      - Less tissue penetration
      - Combination of shorter half-life and decreased tissue penetration results in less myelosuppression than with 89Sr
      - Grade 3–4 neutropenia in less than 10%
      - Grade 3–4 thrombocytopenia in approximately 15%
      - Nadir of 4–5 weeks
      - Said to result in less cumulative bone marrow toxicity
      - Response rates similar to those with 89Sr
    - Rhenium 186 and rhenium 188
      - Beta-emitters
      - High tumor-to-bone marrow accumulation ratio may allow use in patients with compromised bone marrow.

- Nadir of 4–6 weeks
- Toxicity
  - Transient pain flare that may predict response
  - Neutropenia and thrombocytopenia
  - Nadir varies depending on agent
  - Cumulative hematologic toxicity after multiple courses can be significant, particularly in heavily pretreated patients and those with extensive bone involvement.
- Contraindications
  - Acute or chronic renal insufficiency (glomerular filtration rate [GFR], 30 ml/min), as these agents are excreted by the kidneys
  - Severe cytopenias
  - Need for urgent/emergent EBRT (e.g., spinal cord compression)
- Radium 223 (Alpharadin), a highly targeted alpha radiopharmaceutical
- Meta analysis of early Phase 1/2 trials suggested a survival advantage of 29%, improvement in bone pain, and prolonged time to progression for patients receiving Radium 223[52]
  - A large randomized trial ALpharadin in SYMptomatic Prostate CAncer (ALSYMPCA) comparing Radium 223 to placebo (NCT 00699751) was stopped early after a preplanned interim efficacy analysis revealed a survival advantage for Radium 223[53]
    - 922 patients with CRPC with at least two bone metastases and no visceral metastases
    - 2:1 randomization Ra 223 50 kBq/kg q 4 weeks × 6 vs. placebo
    - At about 2 years of follow-up
      - Overall survival was superior (14 mos vs 11.2 months) for Ra 223 compared with placebo. HR 0.695 (95% CI 0.552–0.875 p = 0.00185)

- Time to skeletal related events was longer for Ra 223 compared with placebo (13.6 months vs 8.4 months) HR 0.610 (95% CI 0.461–0.807) p = 0.00046
  * Radium 223 was well tolerated
    - 2% grade 3 or 4 neutropenia
    - 4% grade 3 or 4 thrombocytopenia
  - Based on the results of this trial, FDA approval is expected shortly
  - Some clinicians believe this agent will be the new standard of care for patients with CRPC and bone metastases
  - Radium 223 is the only systemic radioisotope that has shown a survival advantage.
- Conclusion
  * Even though no survival benefit has been demonstrated, systemic radiopharmaceuticals should be considered in patients with multiple painful sites. The use of these agents in combination with chemotherapy is currently under investigation.

■ Surgery

- With the exception of neurosurgery for relief of spinal cord compression (see Chapter 10), or repair of an actual or impending pathological fracture, operative procedures for skeletal metastases have a limited role. Because most prostate cancer metastases are blastic rather than lytic, pathologic fracture of a weight-bearing or long (appendicular) bone is rare.
- Balloon Kyphoplasty is increasingly being used as a less invasive measure for therapy of painful vertebral metastases with compression fracture.[54]

■ Nonspecific Measures

Treatment of General Symptoms of Advanced CRPC

■ Failure to Thrive, or the "Dwindles"

* Low-dose prednisone (10–20 mg/day) has long been known to have a nonspecific beneficial effect on patients with advanced prostate cancer and symptoms such as fatigue, asthenia, anorexia, etc.

■ Pain

* That pain control is important in the management of advanced prostate cancer is axiomatic. The assistance and direct involvement of an expert pain control team is often needed to manage pain in these patients as they inevitably escalate from simple nonsteroidal anti-inflammatory agents, through oral and eventually parenteral opiates, and even more invasive methods.

■ Fatigue (see also Fatigue in Chapter 10)

* Fatigue, one of the most common symptoms reported by patients with advanced prostate cancer, is often the one with the greatest negative effect on quality of life. An attempt should be made to identify the cause of the fatigue (e.g., medication, depression, anemia, metabolic derangements) and treat it accordingly. The value and safety of stimulants such as modafinil in this often elderly population with comorbidities is under investigation.

■ Anorexia

* Anorexia is an extremely disconcerting symptom that may carry with it hidden cultural and existential meanings. As is the case with many symptoms, a diligent search for a correctible underlying cause is required. If no cause is found, pharmacologic intervention should be considered.

  ■ Megestrol acetate (MGA) in doses up to 800 mg/day has been used to treat cancer-related anorexia. Even though this agent was shown to have modest activity against prostate cancer and has been used as second- or third-line hormone therapy, a number of recent reports describe dramatic increases in PSA levels with MGA that normalize after its cessation. Along with concerns about a prothrombotic effect and fluid retention, this has discouraged many oncologists from using this agent. However, for certain patients who are late in their disease course and for whom therapeutic goals are largely palliative, a trial of MGA may result in a very gratifying improvement in appetite and, consequently, quality of life. Under these circumstances, the use of MGA should not be ruled out.

- For patients who are very close to death, loss of appetite and inability to maintain adequate nutrition are common. This often generates requests from patients or their families for more aggressive nutritional support. Once it is explained that this is part of the dying process, patients and their families generally accept this fact and cease requests for more aggressive or invasive means of nutritional support.

- Depression
  - Depression is a common, treatable, and often unrecognized part of the CRPC syndrome. It may be the underlying cause for fatigue, anorexia, and failure to thrive, and it may be responsible for increased tensions between the patient and his loved ones and caregivers. Many men are resistant to interventions aimed at treating depression. However, once depression is explained to the patient as part of the cancer syndrome, similar to pain, anemia, or nausea, most will be more willing to consider antidepressant therapy and/or psychotherapeutic intervention.

■ Complementary Therapy for Prostate Cancer

- The lack of effective therapies for advanced prostate cancer beyond hormones and first-line chemotherapy has driven a large number of patients with AIPC to alternative or complementary approaches. Most of these therapies involve herbal or dietary supplements.
- Dietary additives and modifications
  - Selenium, vitamin E, soy, saw palmetto, and lycopenes are the most commonly used supplements by patients with prostate cancer. Diets that are low in animal fat have also been recommended. Without good data, it

is hard to recommend these as effective complementary approaches specifically for prostate cancer. However, the overall health value of lowering the amount of animal fat in the diet while increasing the amounts of fruits and vegetables justifies their use. It should be emphasized to patients that because the extent of benefits for their prostate cancer is not known, these approaches should not replace standard therapy.

- Herbal compounds
  - PC-SPES
    - PC-SPES is a combination of eight herbal agents that was shown to be effective in CRPC. PSA response rates of greater than 50% were observed in more than 50% of patients in two trials[38,39] with minimal toxicity. In noncastrate patients, serum testosterone levels declined, reinforcing the idea that plant alkaloids with estrogenic function were responsible for the compound's activity. When it was available in the United States (1996–2002), it was widely used. This agent was removed from the market in 2002, when it was found that some lots were contaminated with drugs such as DES, warfarin, indomethacin, and alprazolam. A 2003 trial sought to determine whether PC-SPES had any advantage over DES.[40] In this randomized study, similar activity was found for PC-SPES and DES. However, doubts about the consistency of the production methods and possible contamination with DES make it difficult to draw conclusions.

■ Summary and Conclusions, Treatment of CRPC

- Patients with CRPC should remain on testosterone suppression.
- Chemotherapy may be deferred for patients with biochemical failure alone and for patients with asymptomatic, small-volume metastases.
- Isolated, painful bone metastases can be managed with EBRT in order to delay chemotherapy. However, multiple courses of EBRT or systemic radiopharmaceuticals may make the delivery of subsequent chemotherapy difficult because of cumulative bone marrow toxicity.

- Localized radiotherapy to painful skeletal metastases is sufficiently effective that interruption of chemotherapy is justified.
- Docetaxel-based chemotherapy (q 3 weeks) should be offered to patients with reasonable performance status and adequate bone marrow reserve.
- Patients who experience treatment failure with first-line docetaxel-based chemotherapy and remain in reasonable condition can be offered second-line therapy with cabazitaxel, abiraterone acetate (see Chapter 8), or other agents either currently available or in late stages of testing:
  * Sipuleucel-T
  * MDV 3100
  * ARN 509
  * XL 184
  * Alpharadin
- Adding carboplatin should be considered in patients with high-grade or neuroendocrine-type cancers. Patients with small-cell cancers should be treated as such, with either cisplatin or carboplatin plus etoposide.
- Denosumab should be considered for CRPC patients with bone metastases.
- Systemic radiopharmaceutical therapy should be considered for patients with multiple painful sites.
- Low-dose corticosteroids can be very useful in improving the patient's overall sense of well-being.
- Attention to symptom control, including depression and existential issues, is of immeasurable value.
- Symptom-oriented, supportive care alone is an option that should be discussed with patients whose disease has failed multiple regimens and perhaps even earlier.

■ References

1. Martel CL, Gumerlock PH, Myers FJ, Lara PN. Current strategies in the management of hormone refractory prostate cancer. *Cancer Treat Rev.* 2003;29:171–187.
2. Yagoda A, Petrylak D. Cytotoxic chemotherapy for advanced hormone-resistant prostate cancer. *Cancer.* 1993;71(suppl): 1098–1109.

3. Halabi S, Small EJ, Kantoff PW, et al. Prognostic model for predicting survival in men with hormone-refractory metastatic prostate cancer. *J Clin Oncol.* 2003;21:1232–1237.

4. Smaletz O, Scher HI, Small EJ, et al. Nomogram for overall survival of patients with progressive metastatic prostate cancer after castration. *J Clin Oncol.* 2002;20:3972–3982.

5. Hudes G. Estramustine-based chemotherapy. *Semin Urol Oncol.* 1997;15:13–19.

6. Benson R, Hartley-Asp B. Mechanism of action and clinical uses of estramustine. *Cancer Invest.* 1990;8:375–380.

7. Iversen P, Rasmussen F, Asmussen C, et al. Estramustine phosphate versus placebo as second line treatment after orchiectomy in patients with metastatic prostate cancer: DAPROCA study 9002. Danish Prostatic Cancer Group. *J Urol.* 1997;157:929–934.

8. Loening SA, Beckley S, Brady MF, et al. Comparison of estramustine phosphate, methotrexate and cisplatinum in patients with advanced, hormone refractory prostate cancer. *J Urol.* 1983;129:1001–1006.

9. de Kernion JN, Murphy GP, Priore R. Comparison of flutamide and Emcyt in hormone-refractory metastatic prostatic cancer. *Urology.* 1988;31:312–317.

10. Raghavan D, Cox K, Pearson BS, et al. Oral cyclophosphamide for the management of hormone-refractory prostate cancer. *Br J Urol.* 1993;72(pt 1):625–628.

11. Glode LM, Barqawi A, Crighton F. Metronomic therapy with cyclophosphamide and dexamethasone for prostate carcinoma. *Cancer.* 2003;98:1643–1648.

12. Hussain MH, Pienta KJ, Redman BG. Oral etoposide in the treatment of hormone-refractory prostate cancer. *Cancer.* 1994;74:100–103.

13. Rangel C, Matzkin H, Soloway MS. Experience with weekly doxorubicin (adriamycin) in hormone-refractory stage D2 prostate cancer. *Urology.* 1992;39:577–582.

14. Millikan R, Baez L, Banerjee T, et al. Randomized phase 2 trial of ketoconazole and ketoconazole/doxorubicin in androgen independent prostate cancer. *Urol Oncol.* 2001;6:111–115.

15. Culine S, Kattan J, Zanetta S, Theodore C, Fizazi K, Droz JP. Evaluation of estramustine phosphate combined with weekly doxorubicin in patients with androgen-independent prostate cancer. *Am J Clin Oncol.* 1998;21:470–474.

16. Hudes GR, Greenberg R, Krigel RL, et al. Phase II study of estramustine and vinblastine, two microtubule inhibitors, in hormone-refractory prostate cancer. *J Clin Oncol.* 1992;10: 1754–1761.

17. Seidman AD, Scher HI, Petrylak D, Dershaw DD, Curley T. Estramustine and vinblastine: use of prostate specific antigen as a clinical trial end point for hormone refractory prostatic cancer. *J Urol.* 1992;147(pt 2):931–934.

18. Hudes G, Einhorn L, Ross E, et al. Vinblastine versus vinblastine plus oral estramustine phosphate for patients with hormone-refractory prostate cancer: a Hoosier Oncology Group and Fox Chase Network phase III trial. *J Clin Oncol.* 1999;17:3160–3166.

19. Tannock IF, Osoba D, Stockler MR, et al. Chemotherapy with mitoxantrone plus prednisone or prednisone alone for symptomatic hormone-resistant prostate cancer: a Canadian randomized trial with palliative end points. *J Clin Oncol.* 1996;14:1756–1764.

20. Kantoff PW, Halabi S, Conway M, et al. Hydrocortisone with or without mitoxantrone in men with hormone-refractory prostate cancer: results of the cancer and leukemia group B 9182 study. *J Clin Oncol.* 1999;17:2506–2513.

21. Khan MA, Carducci MA, Partin AW. The evolving role of docetaxel in the management of androgen independent prostate cancer. *J Urol.* 2003;170:1709–1716.

22. Roth BJ, Yeap BY, Wilding G, Kasimus B, McLeod D, Loehrer PJ. Taxol in advanced, hormone refractory carcinoma of the prostate. A phase II trial of the Eastern Cooperative Oncology Group. *Cancer.* 1993;72:2457–2460.

23. Trivedi C, Redman B, Flaherty L, Kucuk O, Du W, Heilbrun L, Hussein M. Weekly 1-hour infusion of paclitaxel. Clinical feasibility and efficacy in patients with hormone refractory prostate carcinoma. *Cancer.* 2000;89:431–436.

24. Petrylak DP. Docetaxel for the treatment of hormone-refractory prostate cancer. *Reviews in Urology.* 2003; 5(suppl 3):S14–S21.

25. Kelly WK, Curley T, Slovin S, et al. Paclitaxel, estramustine phosphate, and carboplatin in patients with advanced prostate cancer. *J Clin Oncol.* 2001;19:44–53.

26. Petrylak DP, Macarthur R, O'Connor J, et al. Phase I/II studies of docetaxel (Taxotere) combined with estramustine in men with hormone-refractory prostate cancer. *Semin Oncol.* 1999;26(suppl 17):28–33.

27. Kreis W, Budman D. Daily oral estramustine and intermittent intravenous docetaxel (Taxotere) as chemotherapeutic treatment for metastatic, hormone-refractory prostate cancer. *Semin Oncol.* 1999;26(suppl 17):34–38.

28. Petrylak DP, Tangen CM, Hussain MH, et al. Docetaxel and estramustine compared with mitoxantrone and prednisone for advanced refractory prostate cancer. *N Engl J Med.* 2004;351:1513–1520.

29. Tannock IF, de Witt R, Berry WR, et al. Docetaxel plus prednisone or mitoxantrone plus prednisone for advanced prostate cancer. *N Engl J Med.* 2004;351:1502–1512.

30. Berry W, Gregurich M, Dakhil S, Hathorn J, Asmar L, US Oncology, Houston, TX. Phase II randomized trial of weekly paclitaxel (Taxol) with or without estramustine phosphate in patients with symptomatic, hormone-refractory, metastatic carcinoma of the prostate [abstract]. *Proc Am Soc Clin Oncol.* 2001;20:175a. Abstract 696.

31. Smith MR, Kaufman DS. Management of bone metastases: external beam radiation therapy, radiopharmaceuticals and bisphosphonates. In: Kantoff PW, Carroll PR, D'Amico AV, eds. *Prostate Cancer: Principles and Practice.* Philadelphia: Lippincott Williams and Wilkins; 2002:595–601.

32. Saad F, Gleason DM, Murray R, et al. Long-term efficacy of zoledronic acid for the prevention of skeletal complications in patients with metastatic hormone-refractory prostate cancer. *J Natl Cancer Inst.* 2004;96:879–882.

33. Estilo CL, Van Poznak CH, Williams T, et al. Osteonecrosis of the maxilla and mandible in patients treated with bisphosphonates: a retrospective study [abstract]. *Proc Am Soc Clin Oncol.* 2004;23:747. Abstract 8088.

34. Neilsen OS, Munro AJ, Tannock IF. Bone metastases: pathophysiology and management policy. *J Clin Oncol.* 1991; 9:509–524.

35. van den Hout WB, Vander Linden YM, Steenland E, et al. Single- versus multiple-fraction radiotherapy in patients with painful bone metastases: cost-utility analysis based on a randomized trial. *J Natl Cancer Inst.* 2003;95:222–229.

36. Pandit-Taskar N, Batraki M, Divgi CR. Radiopharmaceutical therapy for palliation of bone pain from osseous metastases. *J Nucl Med.* 2004;45:1358–1365.

37. Porter AT. Strontium-89 (Metastron) in the treatment of prostate cancer metastatic to bone. *Eur Urol.* 1994;26(suppl 1):20–25.

38. Oh WK, George DJ, Hackman K, Manola J, Kantoff PW. Activity of the herbal combination, PC-SPES, in the treatment of patients with androgen-independent prostate cancer. *Urology.* 2001;57:122–126.
39. Small EJ, Frohlich MW, Bok R, et al. Prospective trial of the herbal supplement PC-SPES in patients with progressive prostate cancer. *J Clin Oncol.* 2000;18:3595–3603.
40. Oh WK, Kantoff PW, Weinberg V, et al. Prospective, multicenter, randomized phase II trial of the herbal supplement, PC-SPES, and diethylstilbesterol in patients with androgen-independent prostate cancer. *J Clin Oncol.* 2004;22:3705–3712.
41. Scher HI, Xiaoyu J, de Bono JS, et al. Circulating tumour cells as prognostic markers in progressive, castration-resistant prostate cancer: a reanalysis of IMMC38 trial data. *Lancet Oncology.* 2009;10:233–239.
42. Scher HI, et al. Circulating tumour cells as prognostic markers in progressive, castraion-resistant prostate cancer: a reanalysis of IMMC38 trial data. *Lancet Oncol.* 2009; 10: 233–239.
43. Berthold DR, Pond GR, Soban F, de Wit R, Eisenberger M, Tannock IF. Docetaxel plus prednisone or mitoxantrone plus prednisone for advanced prostate cancer: updated survival in the TAX 327 study. *J Clin Oncol.* 2008;26(2):242–245.
44. de Bono JS, Oudard S, Ozguroglu M, et al. Prednisone plus cabazitaxel or mitoxantrone for metastatic castration-resistant prostate cancer progressing after docetaxel treatment: a randomised open-label trial. *The Lancet.* 2010; 376 (947):1147–1154.
45. Smith DC, Spira A, De Gre`ve J, et al: Phase 2 study of XL184 in a cohort of patients with castration resistant prostate cancer (CRPC) and measurable soft tissue disease. 22nd European Organisation for Research and Treatment of Cancer-National Cancer Institute-American Association for Cancer Research (EORTC-NCI-AACR) Symposium on Molecular Targets and Cancer Therapeutics, Berlin, Germany, November 16–19, 2010
46. Kelly WK, Halabi S, Carducci MA, et al. A randomized double-blind palcebo controlled phase III trial comparing docetaxel, prednisone and placebo with docetaxel, prednisone and bevacizumab in men with metastatic castration-resistant prostate cancer: survival results of CALGB 90401. [Abstract] ASCO 2010 # LBA 4511.

47. Aggarwal R and Ryan CJ. Castration-resistant prostate cancer: targeted therapies and individualized treatment. *The Oncologist.* 2011; 16: 264–275.

48. Kantoff PW, Higano CS, Shore ND Sipuleucel-T immunotherapy for castration-resistant prostate cancer. *N Engl J Med.* 2010; 363;5:411–422.

49. Garcia JA and Dreicer R. Immunotherapy in castration-resistant prostate cancer: integrating sipuleucel-T into our current treatment paradigm. *Oncology.* 2011; March: 242–249.

50. Fizazi K, Carducci MA, Smith MR, et al. A randomized phase III trial of denosumab versus zoledronic acid in patients with bone metastases from castration-resistant prostate cancer. {Abstr.} ASCO 2010 #LBA4507.

51. Fizazi K, Carducci MA, Smith MR, et al. Denosumab versus zoledronic acid for treatment of bone metastases in me with castration-resistant prostate cancer: a randomized double-blind study. *Lancet Oncology.* 2011; 377:813–822.

52. Nilsson S, Parker C, and Haugen I Alpharadin, a novel, highly targeted alpha pharmaceutical with a good safety profile for patients with CRPC and bone metastases: combined analysis of phase I and II clincal trials. ASCO abstract #106 2010 Genitourinary Cancers Symposium.

53. Bayer's investigational compound radium-223 chloride met its primary endpoint of significantly improving overall survival in a phase III trial in patients with castration-resistant prostate cancer that has spread to the bone. [news release] Wayne, NJ: Bayer HealthCare; June 6, 2011.

54. Berenson J, Pflugmacher R, Jarzem P, et al. Balloon kyphoplasty versus no-surgical fracture management for treatment of painful vertebral body compression fractures in patients with cancer: a multicentre randomized controlled trial. *Lancet Oncology.* 2011; 12:225–235.

CHAPTER 10

Selected Complications of Advanced Prostate Cancer

■ Introduction

Advanced or metastatic prostate cancer is a devastating disease that, while potentially fatal, may evolve over many years. During that time, the patient is vulnerable to a host of complications due to the underlying disease, its treatment, or his other comorbidities. Most, if not all, of these complications are common to all malignancies and thus are well described in the major texts.[1,2] A comprehensive review of this subject is beyond the scope of this handbook. This chapter focuses on only a few of the most common, troublesome, or less well-known problems.

■ Neuropsychiatric Complications

Malignant Spinal Cord Compression (MSCC)

- Spinal cord compression secondary to metastatic prostate cancer is a common complication, one that has a potentially profound negative impact on quality of life, even for patients with limited life expectancy.
- Two publications have comprehensively reviewed the epidemiology, diagnosis, and treatment of MSCC.[3,4] Unless otherwise cited, most of the information in this section comes from these two reviews.
- Incidence
  - Prostate cancer accounts for approximately 20% of all episodes of MSCC.
  - In a population-based study, patients with prostate cancer had a 7.24% cumulative incidence of MSCC in the 5 years preceding death.[5]

- Pathophysiology
  - High incidence of hematogenous dissemination of prostate cancer cells to vertebral bodies
    - The tumor in the vertebral body grows posteriorially, compressing the anterior thecal sac, the epidural vessels, and eventually the spinal cord itself.
  - Bone destruction, less common in prostate cancer, can result in retropulsion of bone fragments and spinal instability.
  - Neurologic deficits can result from direct pressure by tumor, vasogenic edema, spinal cord hypoxia secondary to vascular compromise, or injury due to retro-pulsed bone fragments.
  - MSCC due to intramedullary metastases without bone or epidural involvement is rare.
- Differential diagnosis
  - The differential diagnosis includes
    - Generalized debilitation
    - Leptomeningeal metastases
    - Extrinsic pressure on brain parenchyma from dural metastases
    - Rare intrinsic parenchymal brain metastases
    - Steroid myopathy
    - Pelvic nerve root compression
    - Leg weakness due to painful pelvic bone or node metastases
- Diagnosis of MSCC
  - Maintaining a high index of suspicion is critical, because early diagnosis and treatment are critical in preventing further permanent neurologic damage (see Treatment of MSCC, pp. 237).
  - Every patient with prostate cancer with new or worsening back pain should have a careful history taken, in an attempt to elicit symptoms suggestive of early MSCC, and a thorough neurologic examination.
- Localization[4]
  - Thoracic spine (60–80%)
  - Lumbosacral spine (15–30%)
  - Cervical spine (< 10%)

- Symptoms
  - Back pain is virtually universal.
    - This pain is often described as band-like or as a tightening sensation across the anterior abdomen or thorax.
  - Patients may report abdominal pain alone.
  - 60–85% of patients describe motor weakness or sensory loss.
  - Bowel and bladder dysfunction are usually late-stage phenomena.
  - Ataxia is rare.
  - Patients, particularly those who may be weak and debilitated for other reasons, may not spontaneously offer complaints that would alert the clinician to the possibility of MSCC. The diagnosis should be considered in patients hospitalized for other reasons who remain bedridden and in previously ambulatory outpatients who now need assistance in walking.
- Physical examination may reveal:
  - Motor weakness
  - Sensory loss
  - Abnormal deep tendon reflexes
  - Sustained clonus
  - Extension on plantar reflex (Babinski)
  - If symptoms suggest MSCC, further evaluation should be undertaken, even if the neurologic examination results are completely normal.
- Imaging
  - Magnetic resonance imaging of the spine is the procedure of choice.
    - Sensitivity of 93%
    - Specificity of 97%
  - CT with myelography is commonly used for patients who cannot undergo MRI
- Treatment of MSCC
  - Malignant spinal cord compression is a true oncologic emergency!
  - Early intervention is key in preventing progression of neurologic deficit.

- As many as 70% of patients with MSCC lose some neurologic function between the time symptoms begin and the time treatment is started.[6]
- In general, treatment of MSCC prevents progression rather than reversing functional deficits.
  - Corticosteroids[4]
    - Reduce spinal cord edema
    - Shown to improve outcome when compared with radiotherapy alone.[7]
    - Dose
      - Dexamethasone: 16–100 mg/day
      - No clear-cut benefit for commonly used higher doses
    - Duration of corticosteroid therapy
      - No evidenced-based guidelines
      - Some clinicians recommend that doses should not be tapered until radiotherapy is complete, but toxicity often requires earlier dose reduction.
    - *Note:* Pneumocystis carinii prophylaxis should be considered for patients expected to be on long-term steroid therapy.
  - Radiotherapy for MSCC
    - Unless surgery is planned (see Surgical treatment of MSCC, pp. 239), radiotherapy should be instituted on an emergency basis as soon as the diagnosis is established, including on occasion nights or weekends.
    - Treatment is usually delivered to the site of the MSCC and to 1–2 vertebral bodies above and below it.
      - Doses range from 25–36 Gy in 10–15 fractions.
    - Hypofractionated radiotherapy is becoming more common.

- Results of radiotherapy
  - The likelihood of remaining ambulatory or regaining full ambulatory status depends on the functional status at the time radiotherapy is instituted[8,9] (**Table 10-1**)

Table 10-1 Radiotherapy for Malignant Spinal Cord Compression: Outcome is a Function of Neurological Function at Presentation

Pretreatment Status	Ambulatory after Radiation (%)[8]
Fully ambulatory	93.8
Requires assistance	62.8
Paraparetic	38.0
Paraplegic	12.0

- *Note:* These data refer to patients treated with radiotherapy alone but without bone fragmentation, and include patients with a variety of primary cancers, including some that are highly radiosensitive. The data should be interpreted with these facts in mind. Although patients with prostate cancer rarely have retropulsion of bone fragments contributing to their cord compression, this tumor is less sensitive to radiotherapy than myeloma or multiple lymphoma, for example. Thus, the degree to which paraparetic or frankly paraplegic patients recover may be less than reported in this table.
- Complications of radiotherapy for MSCC
  - Cytopenias
  - Mucositis (after irradiation of cervical spine)
  - Pneumonitis
  - Rare nausea and vomiting
  - Enteritis and, on occasion, bowel obstruction
- Surgical treatment of MSCC
  - Possible indications for surgical management of MSCC
    - Need for tissue diagnosis in patients whose cancers present with MSCC

- Existence of extensive retropulsion of bony fragments
- Spinal instability
- Documented neurologic deterioration during radiotherapy
- MSCC in a maximally irradiated field
- Very rapid evolution of neurologic signs
- Extensive circumferential involvement of the spinal canal

- *Note*: Although there is evidence to suggest that outcomes with surgery are superior to those achieved with radiotherapy alone,[10] surgical treatment of MSCC involves a major procedure in patients who may have limited life expectancy and significant comorbidities. Thus, discretion may be the better part of valor, and considerable judgment should be exercised in deciding the best treatment for any individual patient.
- Laminectomy
  - Surgical removal of the posterior neural arch, allowing decompression of the spinal cord
  - Does not allow for resection of the tumor, usually involving the vertebral body
  - More helpful in less common posterior spinal cord compression
  - Usually followed by radiotherapy (when feasible)
  - *Note*: Although this may be a suboptimal approach compared with anterior decompression, it may be a reasonable compromise for patients in poor condition with limited life expectancy.
- Anterior decompression
  - Surgical procedure of much greater magnitude than laminectomy
  - Requires either thoracotomy or retroperitoneal approach
  - Typically involves resection of the involved vertebral body (bodies) with use of methyl methacrylate and spinal hardware to stabilize the spine

> ▪ Better procedure for patients with unstable spines and extensive bone destruction
> ▪ Should be considered for patients who are in good condition and have a reasonable life expectancy

Base of Skull Syndrome

▪ The propensity for prostate cancer to spread to bone includes the skull. Involvement of the bones of the base of the skull is not an uncommon late-stage phenomenon.
▪ Pathophysiology
  * Cranial nerve palsies due to entrapment at neural foramina
  * May be single or multiple
  * Can involve any cranial nerve
    ▪ Most common cranial nerves involved[11]
      * VI (22%)
      * V (19%)
      * XII (19%)
      * VII (12%)
    ▪ May be limited to smaller subdivisions of cranial nerves
▪ Diagnosis
  * Signs and symptoms[11]
    ▪ Facial numbness
    ▪ Diplopia
    ▪ Tongue deviation
    ▪ Visual loss
    ▪ Aspiration
    ▪ Dysarthria
▪ Imaging
  * MRI or CT of head and skull base
▪ Treatment
  * Radiotherapy and corticosteroids
    ▪ 50% response rate but poor median survival (~3 months)[11]

Depression

▪ Depression is extremely and understandably common among patients with advanced prostate cancer. A detailed discussion of the management of depression is beyond the scope of this handbook. It is mentioned here only because many men are hesitant to admit to being depressed. Therefore, it is up to the clinician to inquire about mood changes and affect. Patients who are resistant to antidepressant therapy and psychotherapy should be led to understand that depression is part of the cancer syndrome and is amenable to treatment.

Fatigue

▪ Fatigue is one of the most common and most vexing problems facing clinicians who care for patients with prostate cancer. This subject is dealt with in the palliative care handbook. Because it is so prevalent in the prostate cancer population, it is briefly discussed here.

▪ Common causes of fatigue
  * Anemia
  * Electrolyte abnormalities and other metabolic abnormalities
  * Inadequate pain control
  * Opiates and other drugs
  * Chemotherapy, AST, and radiotherapy
  * Depression, anxiety, and insomnia
  * Malnutrition
  * Large tumor burden
  * Infection

▪ Management of fatigue[12]
  * Fatigue, like any other symptom, requires a diagnostic evaluation to determine cause when possible, including
    ▪ CBC
    ▪ Electrolytes
    ▪ Chemistries (serum glucose, calcium, creatinine, liver function tests)
    ▪ Thyroid function
  * Correction of what is correctable
    ▪ Transfusion and erythropoietin for anemia

- Adjustment of pain regimen
- Review and adjustment of other medications
- Treatment of depression
- Identification and treatment of concurrent infection
- Use of nutritional supplements
  - The use of megestrol acetate for anorexia in cancer patients is well established. However, progestational agents can cause tumor flare in patients with prostate cancer. These drugs should be used with great caution, and the palliative benefits should be carefully weighed against the risk of worsening the underlying disease.
- Possible intermittent hormone therapy and respite from chemotherapy
- Exercise and psychosocial interventions
- Pharmacologic intervention
  - Methylphenidate
  - Modafinil

■ Hematologic Complications

Cytopenias

- Patients with prostate cancer frequently have chronic anemia and/or thrombocytopenia.
- The etiology of these abnormalities is usually multifactorial and can include:
  - The acute and/or cumulative effect on the marrow of chemotherapy, EBRT, and systemic radioisotope therapy
  - Marrow involvement by prostate cancer cells
  - Concurrent iron, folate, or vitamin B_{12} deficiency
  - Disseminated intravascular coagulation
  - Bleeding, either overt, or occult
- Less commonly, cytopenias may be due to:
  - Autoimmune phenomena associated with cancer
  - Immune cytopenias secondary to drug therapy
  - Alloimmunization after multiple transfusions of either red blood cells (RBCs) or platelets
  - Heparin-induced thrombocytopenia
  - Thrombotic thrombocytopenic purpura

- Management
  - Dependent on cause
  - Transfusion of packed RBCs and platelets as needed
  - Erythropoietin
  - G-CSF for acute and severe chemotherapy- or radio-therapy-induced neutropenia
  - Vitamin B_{12}, folic acid, or iron as indicated

Disseminated Intravascular Coagulation (DIC)[13]

- Bleeding and clotting disorders have long been associated with prostate cancer.
- DIC is seen in two clinical forms—chronic low-grade DIC and acute, fulminant DIC with excessive fibrinolysis.
- Pathophysiology
  - The generation of thrombin, possibly due to tissue factor expressed by tumor cells and endothelial injury, results in intravascular coagulation and consumption of clotting factors. This process, in turn, activates compensatory fibrinolysis. Under normal circumstances, hepatic synthesis of coagulation factors and the presence of fibrinolytic inhibitors keep this process under control. In some cases, for unknown reasons, DIC causes an excessive fibrinolytic state, with potentially catastrophic consequences.
- Chronic low-grade DIC
  - Seen in up to 6–7% of solid tumors
  - Incidence in prostate cancer unknown
  - Characteristics
    - Most common in patients with advanced disease
    - Mild to moderate thrombocytopenia
    - Modest elevation of D-dimer and thrombin-anti-thrombin complex levels
    - Modest prolongation of prothrombin time (PT) and activated partial thromboplastin time (aPTT)
    - Normal or minimally decreased fibrinogen levels
    - Bleeding is uncommon.
  - Management
    - Chronic low-grade DIC generally requires no specific treatment other than therapy of the underlying prostate cancer.

- Fulminant DIC with excessive fibrinolysis[13]
  - Much less common but more dangerous coagulopathy
  - Usually seen in patients with advanced disease
    - Presenting syndrome in rare cases
    - May be precipitated by biopsy of the prostate or of a metastatic site
  - Signs and symptoms
    - Although some patients are asymptomatic, with the diagnosis being made by laboratory abnormalities only, most patients have some form of bleeding, including:
      - Spontaneous skin ecchymoses (**Figure 10-1**)

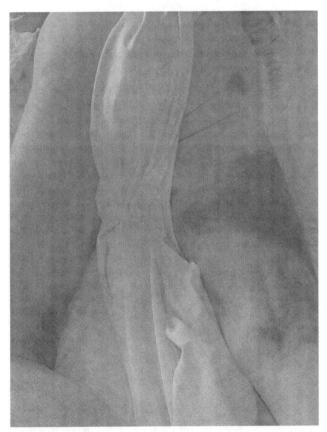

Figure 10-1 Spontaneous skin ecchymoses in a patient with refractory prostate cancer and fulminant DIC. Courtesy of the author.

- Mucosal bleeding
- Hematuria
- GI bleeding
- Retroperitoneal bleeding
- Spontaneous intracranial bleeding (**Figures 10-2** and **10-3**)
- Supratherapeutic international normalized ratio in patients on previously stable warfarin doses
- Laboratory findings
  - Thrombocytopenia may be severe ($< 50,000/mm^3$)
  - Moderate prolongation of PT and aPTT
  - Very high D-dimer levels
  - Serum fibrinogen levels markedly decreased (< 125 mg/dl)
    - It should be remembered that fibrinogen levels are typically elevated in patients with cancer. Thus, even low normal levels of fibrinogen should alert the clinician to the possibility of significant fibrinolysis.

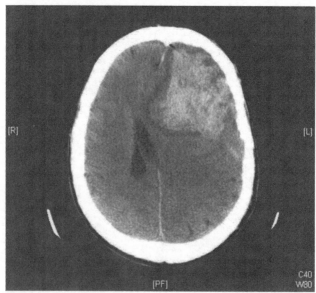

Figure 10-2 Spontaneous intracranial bleeding in a patient with advanced refractory prostate cancer and fulminant DIC. Courtesy of the author.

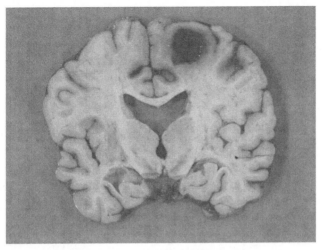

Figure 10-3 Intracerebral hemmorhage in a patient with prostate cancer and DIC. Courtesy of Dr. Mark Edgar.

- ▓ Marked increase in thrombin-antithrombin complex levels
- ▓ Decreased alpha$_2$-antiplasmin levels may precede the drop in fibrinogen
- *Note:* Fulminant DIC with fibrinolysis is an extremely dangerous condition, with a very high risk of fatal intracranial or retroperitoneal hemorrhage that can be sudden and spontaneous. The diagnosis should be entertained, and full coagulation studies should be ordered (including fibrinogen levels), in any patient with prostate cancer and bleeding.
- Management[14]
  - ▓ As always, treat the underlying disease:
    - AST in hormone-naïve patients
    - Estrogens, in the form of IV stilbestrol diphosphate (when available) or via transdermal patch, may exert an antitumor effect and also stimulate the synthesis of clotting factors in the liver.
    - Chemotherapy, even second-line, can result in improvement in coagulation factor levels.

- Replace coagulation factors
  - When fibrinogen levels are below 100 mg/dl, the patient should be given either fresh frozen plasma or cryoprecipitate.
    - Cryoprecipitate is preferable because it is highly concentrated, allowing smaller infusion volumes.
  - Platelet transfusion should be avoided, unless the platelet count is very low (< 10,000/mm^3) or there is major bleeding.
  - The role of factor VII concentrates for major bleeding in the setting of DIC remains to be defined.
- Disruption of the thrombosis/fibrinolysis cycle
  - Low-dose heparin
    - Dangerous in the presence of major hemorrhage
    - Unnecessary in chronic low-grade DIC
  - Antifibrinolytics (tranexamic acid and aminocaproic acid)
    - Used in some centers, but concern that administration of antifibrinolytics will result in unopposed intravascular coagulation makes the use of these agents in fulminant DIC controversial. If DIC is present in addition to fibrinolysis, concurrent use of heparin should be considered.
- *Note*: Beyond treating the underlying disease, the best therapy for cancer-associated DIC remains unknown, as the literature contains only anecdotal reports.

■ Renal and Urologic Complications

- Acute renal failure
  - The diagnosis and management of acute renal failure is extensively discussed in general medicine texts and in major oncology references. For these reasons, the subject is discussed here only as it pertains to patients with prostate cancer.
  - Because prostate cancer is still predominantly a disease of the elderly, antecedent renal dysfunction is not unusual, and susceptibility to new or worsening renal failure is increased.

- The differential diagnosis should also include:
  - Medications
    - Chemotherapy agents typically used for prostate cancer rarely cause renal failure
    - Nonsteroidal anti-inflammatory agents
    - Intravenous contrast media
  - Infection
  - Hypoperfusion secondary to congestive heart failure
  - Acute tubular necrosis
  - Dehydration
    - Dehydration is probably the most common cause of renal failure in patients with prostate cancer. The diagnosis and management of dehydration is usually, but not always, straightforward and is not discussed here.
  - Urinary tract obstruction (UTO)
    - UTO is a very common cause of acute renal failure in patients with prostate cancer. The obstructing lesion can be located at any level of the urinary tract and may be multifocal.
      - Ureteral obstruction due to retroperitoneal or pelvic lymphadenopathy or, less commonly, fibrosis secondary to radiotherapy
      - Outlet obstruction or blockage of the ureteral orifices caused by invasion of the bladder by prostate cancer
      - Obstruction at the level of the prostate due to replacement by cancer, BPH, or stricture
      - Distal obstruction due to invasion of the proximal urethra or penile shaft
    - Nonmalignant obstruction should also be considered.
      - Neurogenic bladder
      - Clot retention
      - Medication (opiates)
      - BPH
      - Stone disease
    - Diagnosis of UTO
      - Foley catheterization to rule out outlet obstruction

- Possible fluid challenge to rule out concurrent dehydration
- Bilateral renal ultrasonography
  - Patients who are dehydrated may not have dilated renal pelves or ureters before volume is replaced.
  - Renal ultrasonography should be repeated after a few days for patients who fail to respond to volume expansion.
- CT urography
- Management of renal failure due to UTO[15]
  - Some patients with outlet obstruction who fail voiding trials may benefit from pharmacologic intervention. Others need palliative TURP or permanent Foley catheterization.
  - For patients with obstruction above the level of the outlet, either internal ureteral stents or percutaneous nephrostomy should be considered.
    - The exact indications and optimal timing of urinary tract stenting remains undefined and highly dependent on the clinical circumstances.
    - Patients with mild hydronephrosis and stable renal function may be observed carefully.
    - On the other hand, the threshold for intervention in patients with preexisting renal disease or only one functioning kidney should be lower.
    - Stents should be considered if chemotherapy with agents excreted by the kidney is anticipated.
  - Internal ureteral stents
    - This involves the cystoscopic placement of semirigid plastic stents.
    - Double-J or pigtail stents are commonly used so that the device is anchored in the renal pelvis and the bladder.

- Advantages
  - Improved patient acceptability (no external devices or collection bags)
  - Easier to maintain
  - Less risk of stent dislodgement
- Disadvantages
  - Requires cystoscopy
  - May not be feasible if ureteral orifices are obstructed or if there is very high-grade obstruction
  - Potential for infection
  - Bleeding, particularly in patients on anti-coagulation therapy
  - Bladder spasm
  - Requires stent exchange every 3–4 months
- *Note*: In general, internal stents are preferable, when feasible, largely because of better patient acceptance.
- Percutaneous nephrostomy
  - Catheter is inserted percutaneously into the dilated renal pelvis and advanced.
  - Advantages
    - Does not require cystoscopy
    - Possibility of internalization exists
  - Disadvantages
    - Higher risk of dislodgement
    - Source of infection
    - Patient discomfort
  - Presence of external tubing may impair sleep
    - Requires more nursing care for maintenance
    - Also requires stent exchange every 3–4 months
- Urinary tract bleeding[15]
  - Urinary tract bleeding is another common complication seen in patients with prostate cancer.
  - Common causes of urinary tract bleeding in patients with prostate cancer
    - Invasion of bladder by tumor
    - Radiation cystitis

- Presence of stents
- Anticoagulation
- Thrombocytopenia
- DIC
- Infection
- Management includes
  - Placement of three-way catheter for bladder irrigation
  - Correction of coagulopathy, when present
  - Antibiotics, if infection present
  - Cystoscopy with fulguration, when conservative management fails
  - Intravesicle therapy not commonly required
    - Bilateral percutaneous nephrostomy sometimes reduces bleeding from the bladder by allowing the bladder to collapse on itself.
    - Hyperbaric oxygen is sometimes used to control bleeding due to radiation cystitis.
      - On rare occasions, cystectomy is needed for intractable bleeding due to radiation-induced cystitis.

■ Metabolic/Endocrine Complications

Hypocalcemia[16]

- Patients with advanced prostate cancer are subject to all the metabolic and endocrine complications that other cancer patients may experience.
  - Hypercalcemia is rare.
  - Hyponatremia due to inappropriate secretion of antidiuretic hormone is fairly common. Because information on the management of this complication is widely available elsewhere, it is not further explored here.
  - Hypocalcemia is somewhat unique to patients with prostate cancer.
- Two unique causes of hypocalcemia in patients with prostate cancer
  - Bisphosphonates
    - The use of bisphosphonates or inhibitors of RANK ligand to prevent osteopenia in patients receiving AST and to relieve pain in patients with manifest osseous metastases is becoming more common.

- Hypocalcemia is occasionally observed after bisphosphonate or denosumab therapy.
  - Hungry bone syndrome
    - Avid deposition of calcium in blastic metastases can lower serum calcium levels.[17]
- Diagnosis
  - Symptoms of neuromuscular irritability may or may not be present.
  - Ionized calcium levels should be determined, because patients with prostate cancer may be malnourished, with decreased serum albumin levels.
  - Primary hypoparathyroidism should be excluded.
- Management
  - Vitamin D and calcium replacement
  - Discontinuation of bisphosphonates should be considered when hypocalcemia is severe.
  - Syndrome of inappropriate antidiuretic hormone (SIADH)
    - Can occur as a result of pain or nausea
    - Patients with small cell cancer of the prostate may have paraneoplastic SIADH.
    - Treatment is correction of underlying cause and fluid restriction.
  - Paraneoplastic Cushing's syndrome[18]
    - More common with small cell cancers of the prostate
    - May not cause typical Cushingoid features
    - More typically signs and symptoms include
      - Hypertension
      - Edema
      - Hypokalemia with alkalosis
    - Treatment
      - Chemotherapy for controlling underlying disease
      - Aldosterone inhibitors
        - Eplerenone preferred over spironolactone which anecdotally may stimulate growth of prostate cancer
      - Bilateral adrenalectomy may be needed in otherwise refractory cases.
      - Other options include ketoconazole or abiraterone acetate.

■ Vascular Complications of Prostate Cancer

Venous Thromboembolic Events

- Thromboembolic events associated with prostate cancer have been observed for almost a century.[13] The expression of prothrombotic proteins by prostate cancer cells, estrogenic therapy (estramustine), stasis secondary to lymph node obstruction, and immobility all contribute to a high risk of venous-thromboembolic events.

- The diagnosis and management of this disorder is also widely discussed in the general medical and oncologic literature. Suffice it to say that emerging data suggest that low-molecular–weight heparin is superior to warfarin in patients with cancer.[19]

Genital and Lower Extremity Edema Syndrome

- Massive genital and symmetrical bilateral lower extremity edema are common and very distressing end-stage phenomena in men with advanced prostate cancer.

- The syndrome is usually due to extensive pelvic cancer.
  - Massive adenopathy
  - Bulky primary tumors

- May be associated with either rectal obstruction or urinary tract obstruction

- Penile edema may interfere with urination, and bladder catheterization may be required.

- Management is difficult.
  - Clot in IVC or in lower extremities should be ruled out or treated if present.
  - Diuretics may offer temporary relief.
    - Because many of these patients are intravascularly depleted due to third spacing, renal function may deteriorate under these circumstances.
  - Elevation of legs and scrotum is recommended.
  - Involved areas should be examined for signs of infectious cellulitis and, if necessary, antibiotics should be started.

- *Note*: This is a very distressing syndrome for patients. They frequently focus on genital or lower extremity edema, even in the face of severe pain and a poor prognosis, commonly requesting diuretic therapy. An explanation as to the cause and the limited therapeutic options is necessary to avoid overtreatment.

■ References

1. De Vita VT, Hellman S, Rosenberg SA, eds. *Cancer: Principles and Practice of Oncology.* 7th ed. Philadelphia: Lippincott Williams and Wilkins; 2005.

2. Kufe DW, Pollock RE, Weichselbaum RR, Bast RC, Gansler TS. Holland-Frei *Cancer Medicine.* 6th ed. Hamilton, ON: ACS-B.C. Decker; 2003.

3. Loblaw DA, Perry J, Chambers A, Laperriere NJ. Systematic review of the diagnosis and management of malignant extradural spinal cord compression: the Cancer Care Ontario Practice Guidelines Initiative's Neuro-Oncology Disease Site Group. *J Clin Oncol.* 2005;23:2028–2037.

4. Prasad D, Schiff D. Malignant spinal-cord compression. *Lancet Oncol.* 2005;6:15–24.

5. Loblaw A, Laperriere NJ, Mackillop WJ. A population-based study of malignant spinal cord compression in Ontario. *Clin Oncol (R Coll Radiol).* 2003;15:211–217.

6. Husband DJ. Malignant spinal cord compression: prospective study of delays in referral and treatment. *BMJ.* 1998; 317:18–21.

7. Sorensen S, Helweg-Larsen S, Mouridsen H, Hansen HH. Effect of high-dose dexamethasone in carcinomatous metastatic spinal cord compression treated with radiotherapy: a randomised trial. *Eur J Cancer.* 1994;30A:22–27.

8. Lovey G, Koch K, Gademann G. Metastatic epidural spinal compression: prognostic factors and results of radiotherapy (in German). *Strahlenther Onkol.* 2001;177:676–679.

9. Maranzano E, Latini P. Effectiveness of radiation therapy without surgery in metastatic spinal cord compression: final results from a prospective trial. *Int J Radiat Oncol Biol Phys.* 1995;32:959–967.

10. Regine WF, Tibbs PA, Young A, et al. Metastatic spinal cord compression: a randomized trial of direct decompressive surgical resection plus radiotherapy vs. radiotherapy alone. *Int J Radiat Oncol Biol Phys.* 2003;57(suppl 2):S125.

11. O'Sullivan JM, Norman AR, McNair H, Dearnaley DP. Cranial nerve palsies in metastatic prostate cancer—results of base of skull radiotherapy. *Radiother Oncol.* 2004;70:87–90.

12. Wagner LI, Cella D. Fatigue and cancer: causes, prevalence and treatment approaches. *Br J Cancer.* 2004;91:822–828.

13. Kampel LJ. Challenging problems in advanced malignancy: Case 2. Disseminated intravascular coagulation in metastatic hormone-refractory prostate cancer. *J Clin Oncol.* 2003;21:3170–3171.

14. Kampel LJ. Thrombotic and hemorrhagic complications of prostate cancer: challenges in diagnosis and treatment. *Pathophysiol Haemo Thromb.* 2003;33(suppl 1):77–104.

15. Johnson EK, et al. Metabolic and endocrine emergencies. In: Yeung SJ, Escalante CP, eds. *Holland-Frei Oncologic Emergencies.* Hamilton, Ontario, Canada: BC Decker; 2002:103–145.

16. Yeung SJ, Lazo-Diaz G, Gagel RF. Metabolic and endocrine emergencies. In: Yeung SJ, Escalante CP, eds. *Holland-Frei Oncologic Emergencies.* Hamilton, Ontario, Canada: BC Decker; 2002:103–144.

17. Szentirmai M, Constantinou C, Rainey JM, Loewenstein JE. Hypocalcemia due to avid calcium uptake by osteoblastic metastases of prostate cancer. *West J Med.* 1995;163:577–578.

18. Hong MK, Kong J, Namdarian B, et al. Paraneoplastic syndromes in prostate cancer. *Nat Rev Urol.* 2010;7:681–692.

19. Lee AY, Levine MN, Baker RI, et al. Low-molecular–weight heparin versus a coumarin for the prevention of recurrent venous thromboembolism in patients with cancer. *N Engl J Med.* 2003;349:147–153.

Index

Note: Italicized page locators indicate photos/figures; tables are noted with *t*.

A

CPSIA information can be obtained at www.ICGtesting.com
Printed in the USA
LVOW070831150312

273209LV00001B/2/P